THE

QUIET PART OUT LOUD

What They Don't Tell You About Somatics, Psychedelics and Trauma

HANS P. ANDERSSEN

The Quiet Part Out Loud

Copyright © 2024 by Hans P Anderssen

Editor: Michelle Robinson

Cover Design: Edge of Water Designs, edgeofwater.com

Interior Formatting and eBook Design: Kailey Salisbury

ISBNs:

Paperback - 978-1-7383696-0-7

eBook - 978-1-7383696-1-4

CONTENTS

NOTE FROM THE AUTHOR

There are many links to online resources referred to throughout the book. These links are important to understanding the concepts under discussion where they appear in the book. At times, the referenced material explains ideas in more detail and is included as an alternative to lengthier text elaborating on these concepts. These links allowed me to add a variety of formats and voices, break up the monotony of text alone, and keep the book shorter.

You will find links to interviews, presentations, TedTalks, animations, song lyrics, published articles, and somatic exercise instructional videos. I would encourage you to take the time to look at these links when they appear in the text to deepen your reading experience.

The e-book provides most convenient access to these resources as the hyperlinks appear within the text of the book. In the print version, the links are listed in the endnotes at the back of the book.

- Hans

ACKNOWLEDGMENTS

Thank you to:

Cascadia Author Services; Kailey Salisbury - Project Manager, Michelle Robinson - Editor, Judith Sanvicente - Marketing; for their professional guidance and assistance in getting this book published.

Matthew Gardner and Anne-Marie Armour - compassionate and wise therapists.

Steve, Derek, Hector, Ingo, James, Nigel, Lloyd and Grant - good friends who have supported and encouraged me.

Most of all; Marisa, Isaac, Jo, Ari, Karsten.

INTRODUCTION

I'm writing a book. I've got the page numbers done.
Steven Wright, comedian

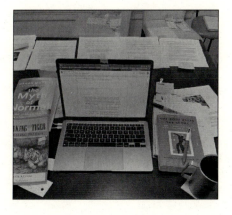

TRUST ME; I'M NOT A DOCTOR

It must be tough to write a book if you're a doctor or an academic. You have to impress your friends, colleagues and peers, you have to use big words, you have to go on and on and on about things in an attempt to convince people that you know what you're talking about, and your book has to be thicker than the other guy's book. Bummer.

I'm neither a doctor nor an academic so I am going to try to keep things short and simple. However, I am big on evidence-based information, research, and the findings and opinions of respected medical and mental health professionals. Therefore, I am going to rely heavily on the writings of a number of specialists who have done all the hard work, in particular three world-renowned experts:

- Peter A. Levine, Ph.D. – the developer of Somatic Experiencing and author of *Waking the Tiger: Healing Trauma*
- Bessel van der Kolk, M.D. – trauma researcher and author of *The Body Keeps the Score: Brain, Mind, and Body in the Healing of Trauma*
- Gabor Maté, M.D. - trauma and addictions specialist, author of multiple books including *When the Body Says No: The Cost of Hidden Stress*, and *The Myth of Normal: Trauma, Illness and Healing in a Toxic Culture*

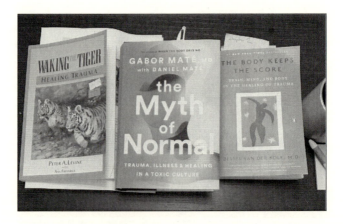

I highly recommend reading - and/or, what I find has additional impact - listening to these books.

PAIN IS FERTILE GROUND

This book was born out of personal experience. Although I had been told for a number of years by multiple therapists that I needed to resolve my trauma and had heard about the benefits of somatics and psychedelics, I was skeptical. As I immersed myself in these modalities for my own well-being, some of what I have come across was so profound and new to me, that I wanted to help get the word out. I don't convey the ideas within this book simply because they are new, intriguing or interesting. I believe they could motivate and encourage those needing and seeking healing. Some of the information could also bring comfort or relief to friends and families of those suffering, and others trying to help them. The ideas that Levine, Maté, van der Kolk and many others are conveying could be life changing - and perhaps lifesaving.

The main underlying ideas behind this book are:

- Trauma is a thing.
- Trauma is held in our bodies.
- Somatics and psychedelics work to resolve trauma.
- Some understated, or unstated, concepts regarding these subjects need to be amplified.

This is most definitely not an exhaustive discussion of these subjects. I focus on a few areas of personal interest to me. It may seem curious that I don't address some topics related to trauma, somatics and psychedelics. Fuller and more complete approaches to these topics are already available elsewhere eg. Maté, Levine and van der Kolk.

I will endeavor to stay in my lane.
My lane:

- Say the quiet part out loud
- Amplify the understated

- Remove barriers to healing and enhance accessibility
- Promote trauma work, somatics, psychedelics and under-utilized modalities
- Direct readers to resources and to do their own research
- Simplify/dumb-down/summarize complex principles
- Use reason and logic to explore outcomes and theories
- Mix in humor, provocation and alternative perspectives
- Yell "he's naked!", when the emperor has no clothes
- Audaciously, unabashedly, shamelessly, brazenly, (and redundantly) quote the experts

Not my lane:

- Pretend to be an expert
- Provide medical or academic explanations
- Regurgitate in detail what experts have already stated elsewhere

TAKING IT FROM WHERE I FIND IT

This book developed organically as I pursued my own healing. Somatics and psychedelics have been, and will continue to be, an important part of my healing journey. I regularly journal, bookmark links, take screenshots, and use my Notes app to record information relevant to my quest. I've taken pictures of the TV screen, sent emails to myself, asked a restaurant server for a pen and napkin, and yelled at Siri while listening to a radio interview to "get this down." After accumulating nuggets, tidbits and crumbs for a couple of years I wondered if some of it may be helpful to other seekers.

In addition to the rich, evidence-based, scholastic writings of Levine, van der Kolk, Maté and others, I draw on a variety of sources including YouTube videos, Facebook posts, Reddit, online discussion forums, conventional and alternative media, inspirational quotes, and memes.

In keeping with the variety of sources, my writing and the format of this book is not conventional. It's quirky, eclectic and perhaps outright weird. While I am dealing with meaty subject matter, it may appear to be delivered in a Spam can. This is both intentional and natural.

I am intentional in avoiding the style and conventions of academics (cuz I ain't one) and traditional authours, in an attempt to stimulate and keep the attention of people like me - those seeking wellness who are tired of obediently trudging through thick conventional tomes.

Secondly, I am a bit quirky and unconventional in nature. I play the accordion, ride a unicycle, and am a big fan of stand-up comedy. But I can also " read a big book", find my way in intellectual dialogue, and I value evidence-based guidance.

I share material that I have come across as I aggressively dug into my own trauma, curiously explored the strange new world of somatics, and daringly experimented with mind-altering psychedelics. I have purposefully left most of what I came across in the format in which I found it. I could have translated or transposed it all into conventional book-ish text, but where possible I chose to leave it in the form in which I was impacted by it.

(*Unfortunately, most images, memes, and screenshots were removed before publication due to copyright laws, but I hope you'll still get the idea*).

My methods of presentation point to some principles that I find valuable, and juxtapose as:

- Rely on experts and specialists - but also be your own guide
- Follow the science - but do your own research
- Set aside focused periods for education - but stay tuned for guidance that comes during the routine and mundane
- Take *your healing* seriously - but don't take *yourself* too seriously

- Do the work - but have some fun
- Teachings and guidance arrive in various forms from diverse sources (*Be alert. The world needs more lerts*)

As far as the somatic practices and exercises that I discuss towards the end of the book go, I will refer to the writings and videos of respected practitioners. This field is new and methodologies and conventions are in development. I endeavor to refer to tools and practices that are common amongst many practitioners and backed either by research or multiple clinical experiences. I have personally tried them all. Don't worry, I'm not going to suggest you stick magnets up your bum or magic stones in your unit. (Although, I haven't actually tried either of those so perhaps I shouldn't pre-judge).

GET PROFESSIONAL HELP

I recommend working under the guidance and oversight of those trained and certified in trauma-informed therapy. However, I do promote self-guidance (see Part 3 - You Are Your Guide) as a supplement to professional therapy. Your situation may be different, but it was impossible for me to find the professional help I needed in some areas in a timely manner. I had to learn about these subjects and practice experimentally on my own. Especially for severe trauma and high-risk symptoms, this may not be advisable.

IT'S ABOUT THE JOURNEY, NOT THE DESTINATION

Substantial parts of this book were built from raw hand-written journal entries. A few years ago I was instructed to write each day as a form of therapy. I had no intention of writing a book. Then I took a writing course, realized I enjoyed it and got some positive feedback. Writing became a creative and somatic outlet for me. I still find writing to be a discipline requiring effort, but this practice provided fulfillment and a sense of accomplishment during a time in my life when I was facing significant challenges and uncertainty. My personal health has improved dramatically by applying the principles in this book.

However, I want to highlight the idea of creating, imagining, and writing about the good, bad and the ugly mid-journey because:

- The medium is the message. Some of the key concepts I convey, such as "it gets worse before it gets better", and "why is this taking so long?", flow from the idea that we are all mid-process. If we think we have to be perfect before we can contribute or be of value, then we all miss out on the treasures each of us hold. I also hope to encourage those suffering to keep going. Never give up. We may never arrive - enjoy the journey.

If you find any succour, relief or helpful guidance in my offering, please know that it comes from - *brace yourself for a nauseating cliche/label* - "a wounded healer".

THEORETICAL OR THERAPEUTIC

Here at the beginning, and again at the end of this book, I am going to suggest something to the reader: radical skepticism. As you study messages of hope from Maté, van der Kolk, Levine, and other experts, challenge them to convince you. Are they cruelly over-promising, or humbly understating? The message they carry is either beautiful or brutal. Those seeking relief should feel free to ask the hard questions:

- Does this stuff really work?
- Are these fluffy theories, or fulsome therapies?
- Are these offerings prophetic or pathetic?

I have the utmost respect, admiration and gratitude for these scholars and teachers. I believe that they are motivated by compassion and a desire to relieve suffering. These world-renowned trauma specialists have devoted their lives, put their reputations on the line, and offered some big ideas:

- Everybody has trauma
- Trauma is trapped in our bodies
- Healing is possible
- Somatics and psychedelics can facilitate healing.

Those who are desperate for healing, and aggressively trying to get better, are not looking to play games and chase after hints, hype and half-baked remedies. We are not content to be offered myths as we desperately search for solid answers.

Are these specialists offering a possible solution? For many, these are life or death questions and we need to be honest with ourselves, as well as with those who offer solutions.

Maté, Levine and van der Kolk have devoted their careers to these subjects. They are either heroes or zeros. Only a zero would offer broken oxygen masks to those of us gasping for air. But a person of compassion who has spent their life seeking to help the trauma sufferer would throw out a potential lifeline, even if the outcome is not guaranteed. I believe these men offer us lifelines. But don't take my word for it.

(*Yes, I mixed metaphors. Yes, I'm leaving it like that.*)

SOME WORKING DEFINITIONS

Trauma

A simple way of defining trauma is that it's an overwhelming experience. Because it exceeds what we were meant to handle, it leaves an imprint in one's nervous system, body, and psyche. It shows up in multiple forms of illness or challenging symptoms.

Traumatic events can occur early in life, or later. They can occur slowly over time, such as in an oppressive parental relationship, or suddenly, as in a serious accident or assault.

Traumatic events can be difficult to define because the same event may be more traumatic for some people than for others.

Somatics

Somatics describes any practice that uses the mind-body connection to help you survey your internal self and listen to signals your body sends about mental and emotional issues, as well as areas of pain, discomfort, or imbalance.

Somatics can be used to describe a variety of forms of movement and healing modalities. Pretty much any type of movement or therapy that involves paying attention to your internal physical sensations and experiences can be described as somatic. These practices allow you to access more information about the ways experiences are held in the body. This information, combined with movement and touch, can facilitate healing and wellness.

There are a wide range of practices, and no strict definition of what is somatic and what is not. Some common practices include yoga, breath-work, Pilates, eye-movement, dance, and massage; but there are many more.

Psychedelics

Psychedelics, sometimes called psychoactive drugs or, when appropriate, psychoactive plants, are drugs whose primary effect is to trigger non-ordinary mental states and an expansion of consciousness. They generally cause specific psychological, visual, and auditory changes, and oftentimes a substantially altered state of consciousness. They have been used beneficially by many cultures throughout history.

Scientific research is providing significant evidence of their effectiveness for a variety of purposes.

Experts agree that psychedelics will soon be part of mainstream Western medical practice.

Note: It has become clear to me that people get weird very quickly when the topic of psychedelics comes up. I'll provide more detail later but here are some initial comments to set the tone regarding my approach to psychedelics:

- My limited therapy so far, all under the guidance of trained therapists, has included psilocybin, lysergic acid diethylamide, ayahuasca and 5-MeO-DMT. There are many other effective medicines. Information and resources related to them are abundant.
- Regarding these substances, I am neither an expert, ecstatic, nor evangelist.
- I do not take the use of psychedelics lightly or trivially. My approach to these medicines has been one of skepticism and caution.
- I am not promoting recreational use and superficial applications. I am focused on serious intention, therapeutic use and mental health benefits.
- My treatments were brief and intensive. They took place over a total of 10 days over a 2 year period. I am neither dependent on nor under their influence during daily life.
- I do not believe these medicines would have been effective as a stand-alone treatment for me. They were a key element, but only as one part of lengthy, multi-faceted therapy.

PART ONE
TRAUMA

CHAPTER 1
EVERYONE HAS TRAUMA

"Trauma has become so commonplace that most people don't even recognize its presence. It affects everyone."
– Peter Levine, *Waking the Tiger*

"It is hard to imagine the scope of an individual life without envisioning some kind of trauma, and it is hard for most people to know what to do about it."
– Mark Epstein, *The Trauma of Everyday Life*

Does everyone have trauma? Do you have trauma? Perhaps the reason you are reading this book is because, like I did two years ago, you are asking yourself, "do I have trauma?"

This book is based primarily on the writings of three world-renowned trauma researchers, Bessel van der Kolk, Peter Levine and Gabor Maté. Their writings on this subject are voluminous. Here is a summary statement from each of them suggesting that we all have some degree of trauma:

"Trauma happens to us, our friends, our families, and our neighbors."
– Bessel van der Kolk, The Body Keeps the Score
(pg. 1)

"Each of us has had a traumatic experience at some time in our lives, regardless of whether it left us with an obvious case of post-traumatic stress."
– Peter Levine, Waking the Tiger (pg. 41)

"There are very few who aren't traumatized. Very few."
– Gabor Maté, "Dr. Gabor Maté Answers the Question: Is Everyone Traumatized?" | A *Mindspace* Podcast Clip[1]

Interestingly, all three of these famous researchers and authors provide detail about their own personal trauma stories. Each one is quite different from the other. Their experiences land at different points across the broad spectrum of trauma:

In *The Body Keeps the Score*, Bessel van der Kolk recounts how he arrived for his first EMDR training in need of some trauma processing himself. He had recently suffered back-to-back losses of clinics, colleagues, and resources.

"It might have all been a coincidence, but it felt as if my whole world was under attack."
– Bessel van der Kolk, The Body Keeps the Score
(pg. 253)

In an interview series sponsored by *PsychAlive*, which you can watch on YouTube, Peter Levine recounts his personal traumatic experience of being hit by a car and allowing the shock to pass out of his body with the reassuring presence of other bystanders.

"Of course, I had no idea how seriously injured I was, no idea."

– Peter Levine, "Dr. Peter Levine on Working through a Personal Traumatic Experience"[2]

Gabor Maté has had his own experiences with trauma from a very young age, being born to a Jewish family shortly before Nazi Germany invaded Budapest. You can hear him speak more about his experiences in an interview on The Chris Hedges Report.

"So I spent the first year under predictably difficult, even life-threatening circumstances, which culminated with my mother giving me to a total stranger in the street in Budapest, because where we were living, I would not have survived."

– Gabor Maté, "Dr. Gabor Maté on Trauma, Addiction, and Illness under Capitalism" | The Real News Network[3]

SO WHAT?

I suppose that if we accept the fact that most if not all of us have trauma, we can respond in one of two ways:

Option one is to explore the possibility that we may have experienced trauma, we gain awareness of symptoms in our own lives, and we can begin to resolve our trauma.

The second option would be to conclude, "well if everyone has trauma, it doesn't seem to be bothering most people - they seem just fine. No one I know is doing anything about their trauma - it doesn't need to be a big deal for me either."

I suggest the first approach may be the healthiest response - for us, our families, and our communities.

GOOD NEWS!

And now the good news - Peter, Bessel and Gabor assure us that trauma can be healed:

"Trauma is a fact of life. It does not, however, have to be a life sentence. Not only can trauma be healed, but with appropriate guidance and support, it can be transformative."
– Peter Levine, *Waking the Tiger* (pg. 2)

"This vast increase in our knowledge about the basic processes that underlie trauma has also opened up new possibilities to palliate or even reverse the damage. We can now develop methods and experiences that utilize the brain's own natural neuroplasticity to help survivors feel fully alive in the present and move on with their lives."
– Bessel van der Kolk, *The Body Keeps the Score* (pg. 3)

"Healing is not guaranteed, but it is available. It is no exaggeration to say at this point in Earth's history that it is also required. Everything I have seen and learned over the years gives me confidence that we have it in us."
– Gabor Maté, *The Myth of Normal* (pg. 11)

So although we have all been affected by trauma, we have the potential to heal; through curiosity, hope, perseverance, and a little help from others. Healing is not guaranteed, but it is available.

CHAPTER 2
THE SYMPTOMS OF TRAUMA

"If you are experiencing strange symptoms that no one seems able to explain, they could be arising from a traumatic reaction to a past event that you may not even remember. You are not alone. You are not crazy. There is a rational explanation for what is happening to you."
– Peter Levine, *Waking the Tiger* (pg. 5)

In his book *Waking the Tiger*, Peter Levine lists 38 symptoms of trauma. For me, reading three pages of symptoms kind of blunts the pointy impact, ie. if everything is attributable to trauma, then so what? Throwing the trauma blanket over everything seems on one hand kind of suffocating, and on the other like an over-simplification.

But perhaps another take-away is to consider that many of our challenges may be rooted in past overwhelming experiences, relationships, or periods of high stress. Some of the more common symptoms from Levine's lists are:

- Anxiety
- Mood swings
- Depression

- Difficulty sleeping
- Fears and phobias

Additionally, I will highlight a particularly troubling and common symptom:

"Addiction is always rooted in childhood trauma and the addiction is an attempt to deal with the effects of childhood trauma which it does temporarily while creating more problems in the long term."
– Gabor Maté, "How Childhood Trauma Leads to Addiction" | *After Skool* [1]

More on the subject of trauma and addiction later.

SIRI, WHAT'S ANOTHER WORD FOR TRAUMA?

Trauma is an overused term that turns people off and prevents them from addressing significant issues and moving forward in their healing. For many years I had a general idea that there were some unhealthy dynamics in my past that may have lingering effects, but it wasn't until I was 50 that a psychologist diagnosed me with significant unaddressed trauma. Additionally, he stated that I was ignorant to the impacts of it, and that it would take extensive work to address it.

Even after seeing the doctor's diagnosis in black and white, for years I was reluctant to do anything about it because:

- It felt whiny and narcissistic to admit I had trauma,
- I had embedded personal and societal stigmas and stereotypes,
- Others had experiences that were worse than mine,
- I thought I should be able to get over it,
- It was a long time ago,

- None of my friends seemed to be affected by trauma, talked about it, or were seeking help for it,
- I had no clue how to get better

The pivotal moment when I decided to address my trauma occurred years later after many diagnostic sessions with a particular therapist (there were many others before her). Picking up on my ambivalence, ignorance and resistance, she provided me with some clear guidance.

I recall her leaning forward in her chair, looking me in the eyes, and talking in a compassionate but deadly serious tone. It reminded me of a doctor with lab reports in hand conveying the diagnosis and treatment for a deadly disease:

1. Hans, you have experienced trauma and you need help with it.
2. You do not need others to confirm, validate, verify or understand your trauma.
3. You do not need to justify or explain your trauma to doubters or skeptics.
4. The same experience can be traumatizing for one person, and not for another.
5. Everyone experiences trauma differently.
6. You have a lot of work to do. Get on with it.

For some reason, the therapist's words impacted me deeper than in past trauma counseling sessions, and I decided to be intentional and aggressive in pursuing healing.

The last few years have been quite a journey and I have been surprised to discover fundamental pieces of information that are understated, hidden or not well communicated. I hope to simplify and amplify these concepts in an effort to help and motivate others to not give up on their pursuit of freedom.

WHAT IS TRAUMA?

Definitions and detailed scientific explanations abound. I encourage you to do some digging around this subject on your own. As I repeat multiple times, I avoid providing detailed psychoneuroimmunological explanations because:

- Detailed information is readily available elsewhere (e.g. Maté, van der Koch, Levine).
- Researching, studying and discovery can be part of one's self-guided healing process.
- I am not an expert.

Here are a few definitions of trauma:

"Trauma is a psychic wound that leaves a scar. It leaves an imprint in your nervous system, in your body, in your psyche, and then shows up in multiple ways that are not helpful to you later on."
– Gabor Maté

"Trauma is a term used to describe the challenging emotional consequences that living through a distressing event can have for an individual. Traumatic events can be difficult to define because the same event may be more traumatic for some people than for others.

However, traumatic events experienced early in life, such as abuse, neglect and disrupted attachment, can often be devastating. Equally challenging can be later life experiences that are out of one's control, such as a serious accident, being the victim of violence, living through a natural disaster or war, or sudden unexpected loss."
– Center for Addiction and Mental Health

"The simplest way of defining trauma is that it's an experience we have that overwhelms our capacity to cope."

– Dr. Dan Siegel, clinical professor of psychiatry at the UCLA School of Medicine

Bessel van der Kolk, M.D., defines trauma as "not the story of something that happened back then, but the current imprint of that pain, horror, and fear living inside the individual".

I agree with Sukie Baxter who states, "I don't actually like the word trauma" (By the way, the YouTube video "How to Release Trauma Stored in the Body"[2] in which Sukie Baxter makes this statement, is amazing. It's only 10 minutes and packed full of great information - I highly recommend it).

She goes on to talk about the need to discharge stress from our bodies. This is very much in line with what Gabor Maté talks about in *When the Body Says No*. He refers his readers to Hans Selye, sometimes called "the father of stress" (my sons might have someone else named Hans in mind).

Selye promoted the idea of various levels or degrees of stress; while we often view stress as being negative, Selye discusses eustress. "Eu" is the Greek prefix for good, so eustress means good stress. At the other end of the spectrum is distress, or stress which we are not designed or able to cope with - in other words, trauma.

Thinking along a continuum of stress is helpful. When the stress is at a level that is overwhelming, it is at a traumatic level. A common phrase in the trauma world combines the use of both words stress and trauma; Post Traumatic Stress Disorder, and the word stress will often mix into specialists' writing about trauma.

Trauma specialists agree that there are gradations or a variety of levels of trauma. I would suggest it is appropriate to think of trauma as "an overwhelming level of stress". This perspective lends itself to understanding that what is an overwhelming level of stress for one person may not be overwhelming for someone else.

SOME TYPES OF TRAUMA

Note: Not an exhaustive list!

Trauma in Utero

"The emotional needs not being met has direct, and defined, and definable physiological effects on the brain and the body. And this begins in utero."

- Gabor Maté, "Dr. Gabor Maté on the Effects of Trauma During Pregnancy and Childhood on Human Development" | *Mindspace*[3]

Intergenerational Trauma

(See more on this later in the chapter)

"Trauma is not just personal, it's cultural, historical and it's also transgenerational. We just can't help passing it on. So, if I carry trauma, I can be sure to pass it on to my kids - unless I've resolved it and worked it out."

– Gabor Maté, "Dr Gabor Maté: Transgenerational Trauma, Stressed Environment, and Child's Diagnosis | *IoPT Norway*[4]

Self-Caused Trauma

I make this distinction because trauma is often seen as coming from an event or experience that was external to us or caused by a person other than ourselves. However, I have become aware that some of my personal decisions and actions have had traumatizing effects and left disastrous impacts - on myself and others.

Many of us regret actions or behaviors from the past and may carry a deep sense of guilt or shame. I would suggest that regret and shame can manifest as overwhelming stress. These self-caused traumas require resolution just as much as those perpetrated by others.

Practicing self-awareness, self-forgiveness, self-compassion, seeking resolution with myself and others, and learning to release this trauma emotionally, psychologically and physiologically can be a key part of our journey.

Dormant Trauma

"The symptoms of trauma can be stable (ever-present), unstable (they will come and go), or they can hide for decades."
– Peter Levine, *Waking the Tiger* (pg. 149)

For many of us, the source or cause of the trauma wounds occurred far in the past and we may not connect them to the glaring issues that are manifesting many years later. It was profoundly helpful to learn that the radical decline in my health occurring in my 40's and 50's was connected to, in part, events from decades earlier.

To be clear, there were absolutely some circumstances in my midlife years that triggered the symptoms of trauma. The trauma that had been trapped in my body for years, was added to throughout my life, and finally re-energized or manifested in recent years. Some re-traumatizing events had stirred up old wounds and "awoke the beast".

"Because trauma symptoms can remain hidden for years after a triggering event, some of us who have been traumatized are not yet symptomatic."
– Peter Levine, *Waking the Tiger* (pg. 41)

Slow Trauma vs Fast Trauma

Trauma incurred gradually over a long period can be just as damaging as a sudden traumatic event. Systemic psychological or emotional trauma within a family, systemic racism, religious system or a spousal relationship can be crippling. Yet it can be difficult to identify, challenge and break free from this more subtle yet insidious form of sustained stress.

Some other forms of trauma (again, this is not meant to be an exhaustive list - there are many other sources and publications):

Trauma in Infancy
Childhood Trauma
Acute Trauma
Sustained/Prolonged Trauma
Chronic Stress
Psychological Trauma

EVERYONE IS IMPACTED DIFFERENTLY

"An experience that's traumatizing for one person may not be traumatizing to another. I think that's really what the research is telling us ... So, people can have different contexts where something that would be traumatizing for you wouldn't be traumatizing for me. ... It's different from anything you've ever experienced before, and in that sense, it overwhelms your ability to cope."
– Dan Siegel, MD

Because trauma is so broad, and such a universal experience, it manifests in many different ways. Trauma is different for each person: it affects us differently, and we recover from it differently. Being aware of this will help us to face and resolve our own trauma, and to be less judgemental of others struggling with the symptoms of trauma.

CHAPTER 3

TRAUMA IS STORED IN YOUR BODY

"Now what we have with trauma is we have his tremendous excitation, and then, boom, we're overwhelmed. This energy becomes locked - it becomes stuck in our bodies."
– Peter Levine, "Peter Levine Demonstrates How Trauma Sticks in the Body" | *PESI*[1]

That trauma is stored in my body was a radical and mind-blowing idea for me.

Emotions get trapped in the body after something traumatic happens to us and the nervous system stays stuck in survival mode. While stuck in this state, stress hormones continue to surge through our bodies even though the event is over. When the body is under this constant level of stress, physical and psychological symptoms emerge.

I am not going to provide extensive information on this subject, because I am not an expert and quite frankly, I don't fully understand the psychoneuroimmunology behind trauma and somatic experiencing. I am not suggesting I am totally ignorant, but I rely on the training and knowledge of medical and therapeutic specialists to understand the scientific complexities.

For example, seven years ago I was diagnosed with atrial fibrillation that required ablation surgery. I gained some understanding of my condition, as well as the ablation procedure, but I was content to trust that my doctors were educated and fully prepared to fix my ticker. I carry a similar level of reliance on the expert's opinion that trauma is stored in our bodies.

By not providing a detailed analysis and explanation, it may appear I am under-valuing the importance of the idea of trauma being stored in our bodies. But the opposite is true. It was essential for me to understand, or at least believe that there was a purpose to me doing somatics. If trauma was not stored in my body, then there was little or no point in doing body work to resolve it.

I became convinced that trauma was trapped or stored in my body, which enabled me to intentionally and even aggressively go after it. If I didn't have the underlying belief that my symptoms could be diminished and I could resolve my trauma by doing these new alternative treatments, then I wouldn't have done them.

Fortunately, and thankfully, this early belief and trust in what the specialists were saying has brought about significant change. The theoretical has become experiential. Doing somatics - bodywork, movement, and physical activities with intention and awareness, can unlock these emotions and facilitate healing.

"Traumatic symptoms are not caused by the "triggering" event itself. They stem from the frozen residue of energy that has not been resolved and discharged; this residue remains trapped in the nervous system where it can wreak havoc on our bodies and spirits."
– Peter Levine, *Waking the Tiger* (pg. 19)

"The body keeps the score: If the memory of trauma is encoded in the viscera, in heartbreaking and gut-wrenching emotions, in autoimmune dis-orders and skeletal/muscular problems, and if mind/brain/visceral

communication is the royal road to emotion regulation, this demands a radical shift in our assumptions."
— Bessel van der Kolk, *The Body Keeps the Score* (pg. 88)

"No matter how sophisticated our minds may be, the fact remains that their basic contents - what we think, believe consciously or unconsciously, feel or are prevented from feeling - powerfully affect our bodies, for better or worse."
— Gabor Maté, *When the Body Says No* (pg. 45)

An article[2] in the online magazine Medium.com informs us of the impacts on the brain and the body and the increased risk of mental and physical problems:

"The truth is that trauma is not just "in your head" ... The emotional and physical reactions it triggers can make you more prone to serious health conditions including heart attack, stroke, obesity, diabetes, and cancer, according to Harvard Medical School research."[3]

So, as you can see, trauma is not merely a phenomenon that is "all in your head." It is stored in your body, and manifests itself as physical symptoms. As such, both body and mind must be taken into account for recovery.

CHAPTER 4
FAMILY

"It has been transformative for me to realize that my own mental health issues carry genuine meanings that arose from my life within my family of origin in a particular historical context."
— Gabor Maté, *The Myth of Normal* (pg. 256)

And I will die in the house that I grew up in.
I'm homesick.
Noah Kahan - Homesick (Official Lyric Video)[1]

NO PERFECT FAMILIES

"Nobody grows up under ideal circumstances - as if we even know what ideal circumstances are."
— Bessel van der Kolk, *The Body Keeps the Score* (pg. 306)

Trauma caused by overwhelming stress or dysfunction (an overused word that has lost its punch) within family systems has some unique and insidious characteristics:

> 1. A child tends to assume that their family system is normal. It is all they know. The victim does not have an objective perspective. How does a child measure their family environment against a healthy one? Therefore there is little opportunity to defy, voice complaints or oppose the system. Instead, damage to the tender mind-body occurs with little resistance, and maladaptive behaviors and crippling symptoms manifest.

"Unlike adults, they have no other authorities to turn to for help - their parents are the authorities. ... Children are also programmed to be fundamentally loyal to their caregivers, even if they are abused by them."
– Bessel van der Kolk, *The Body Keeps the Score* (pg. 135)

> 2. Sustained, long-term abuse is not as identifiable as a temporal traumatic event. Systemic stress, neglect and abuse is not as apparent.

The in-the-moment terror and ongoing suffering from a singular event such as physical or sexual abuse is horrific. The pain is exacerbated by the fact that the event occurred at a particular time and place. These markers frame the moment in a dark and heavy memory.

However, trauma incurred gradually but severely over years can be less easy to identify. It is like the slow torturous drip of a tap, compared to the deluge of pain incurred in a singular event. But day by day, word by word, the torture continues and the damage is done.

Therapist Emmylou Antonieth Seaman, in a recent article in the

Hindustan Times titled "Key Signs of Childhood Emotional Neglect" states:

"The absence of emotional support during childhood can be just as harmful and long-lasting as other traumatic experiences. However, because it's not easy to pinpoint when and where the emotional wounds occurred, it can be challenging to recognise and overcome them."

3. Mental and emotional abuse such as manipulation, control and fear can be just as damaging as physical or sexual abuse.

"If you come from an incomprehensible world filled with secrecy and fear, it's almost impossible to find words to express what you have endured."
– Bessel van der Kolk, *The Body Keeps the Score*
(pg. 298)

BOTH SIDES OF THE COIN

Van der Kolk shares the dramatic family processing experience of a participant named Maria during PBSP psychomotor group therapy. First she describes the beatings that her mother, as well as her and her siblings, endured. She grew up believing that her family, and the lingering sense of fear that filled their home, was normal.

But that sense of fear wasn't all-encompassing; her memories of her mother were loving and warm, comforting in response to her father's rage. Looking back on the events as an adult, she realized that her mother must have felt a lot of fear as well, and the sensation of being trapped.

Maria states:

"'My sadness goes out to my mom; how incapable she was of standing up to my father and protecting us.'"

– **Bessel van der Kolk,** *The Body Keeps the Score*
(pg. 305)

THEY DID THE BEST THEY COULD

I was touched by Maté's exploration of his own role as a father. It caused me to think of my father, and also, from a personal sense of responsibility, of the marks I have left on my four sons:

"However noble our intentions, our ability to carry them out is heavily influenced by our own early experiences and unresolved traumas, by the social expectations we are charged with transmitting to our children, and by the stresses of life."
– **Gabor Maté,** *The Myth of Normal* **(pg. 180)**

As much as we may try, our own unhealthy dynamics or household stress can become a source of trauma for our children, just as they were a source of trauma for us. We do well to gain awareness, accept responsibility, and do our best to mitigate it, for our sake as well as theirs.

To my boy, my precious gentle warrior
To your sweetness and your strength in exploring
May this bond stay with you through your days
My mission is to keep the light in your eyes ablaze
Alanis Morissette: "Ablaze"[2]

CHAPTER 5
INTERGENERATIONAL TRAUMA

"Trauma is not just personal, it's cultural, historical and it's also transgenerational. We just can't help passing it on. So, if I carry trauma, I can be sure to pass it on to my kids - unless I've resolved it and worked it out."
– Gabor Maté, "Dr Gabor Maté: Transgenerational Trauma, Stressed Environment, and Child's Diagnosis | *IoPT Norway*[1]

In the video "Cultivating Transgenerational Resilience: Healing Ancestral Trauma"[2], Dr. Arielle Schwartz provides some fascinating insights based on her professional work, but also includes remarkable references to her experience of exploring her own ancestry.

We are affected by the trauma of past generations occurring before birth and conception.

I am not going to go into detail on this subject - again, I will leave that to the researchers and experts. I broach this subject for two reasons:

1. To facilitate healing by creating awareness of ancestral trauma.

2. To set the stage for a later discussion where I will flip this concept on its head and situate it in perhaps a more positive or solution-oriented light; transgenerational somatics as a healing modality - see Part 4.

On the simplest level, the concept of intergenerational trauma acknowledges that exposure to extremely adverse events impacts individuals to such a great extent that their offspring find themselves grappling with their parents' post-traumatic state.

A more recent and provocative claim is that the experience of trauma – or more accurately the effect of that experience – is "passed" somehow from one generation to the next through epigenetic mechanisms affecting the DNA or genes.

All it takes is one person heroically shielding their child from past generations' trauma to break the cycle. And there are plenty of illustrations, memes and other visualizations to be found portraying just that: with past generations spouting negativity, and just one person in the chain refusing to do the same. They may not be able to accomplish more than that, but it creates the opportunity for the next generation to be even better and say positive things to their children instead.

One illustration I came across showed 5 people in an intergenerational chain; great-great- grand-father, great-grandfather, grandfather, then father and child. The eldest 3 were all yelling harsh abusive words at their child, but the fourth man, the father, had broken the chain and was saying loving words of affirmation to his child.

This portrayal may seem a bit over-dramatic and perhaps displaying something simplistic or harmless. I mean, what's the big deal, can a few words really hurt someone that badly? Well, yes they can. Statements like this from a parent land on the child as determinative proclamations. They become fire-branding, crippling characterizations.

Additionally, parental verbal abuse rarely stands alone. It is most often only one part of a bulging sinister package; psychological abuse, emotional abuse, lack of attunement, affection and affirmation etc.

One key point is that trauma is perpetuated. Another one is a positive message: There is an opportunity to break the cycle.

For transgenerational trauma that has mutated our genes and is imprinted within the body, my understanding is that the work will not be easy. But can we not hope, try, and persevere?

Accepting that intergenerational trauma is actually a thing is not about blaming others or side-stepping personal responsibility. Gaining understanding of these principles compels us to do the hard work of healing and transformation. Turning on the light-switch in the dark, messy attics of our parents, grandparents, and ancestors allows us to begin the process of sorting, discarding and cleaning.

CHAPTER 6
ADDICTION AND TRAUMA

"Because it is all about trauma."
– Gabor Maté

G abor Maté worked for decades in Vancouver's downtown eastside. Through his writings, interviews, seminars, classes and videos, Gabor Maté has been tirelessly providing scientific proof and research to back up the message that addiction is a symptom of trauma.

In the informative video, "The REAL Cause of Drug Addiction ... and a Plant Medicine Solution"[1], he once again succinctly summarizes the link between trauma and addiction:

"Don't ask the question, 'why the addiction?' But, 'why the pain?' ... Addiction is a response to suffering, and what people need in response to addiction is not judgment and simply symptom control; they need to be helped to heal from their trauma."

A widely used tool for measuring trauma incurred during childhood was based on a study in the 1990's into Adverse Childhood

Experiences, now known as the ACE study. More than fifty thousand patients were evaluated annually for a number of years. The researchers developed ten questions that trauma therapists commonly ask during the initial assessment of their client's trauma which enable them to rate trauma on a scale of one to ten. In The Body Keeps the Score, van der Kolk reports:

> *"The ACE study revealed that traumatic life experiences during childhood and adolescence are far more common than expected."*

And later, he cites the strong correlation between a high ACE score (i.e. higher levels of childhood trauma) and substance abuse: that people with a middling ACE score (4-7) were 7x more likely to identify as alcoholics than those with an ACE score of 0; and that people with a high ACE score (6+) had a 4,600% greater likelihood to use injection drugs than those with a score of 0.

Gabor Maté has been attempting to hammer home the correlation between trauma and addiction for decades. He collaborated with After Skool to create an 11-minute animated video, How Childhood Trauma Leads to Addiction[2], which I think communicates the basics of this undeniable connection clearly and concisely. I highly recommend checking it out.

CHAPTER 7
TRAUMA, DRAMA, CRY TO YOUR MOMMA

I have a love/hate relationship with this trauma stuff. I do not like to admit that there is something in my past that hinders me, and I can't just "get over it" or ignore it, as I feel I should be able to do.

I realize that much of the skepticism and criticism around my trauma and doing trauma work comes from within. Imaginary critics offer their observations:

- He's just avoiding taking personal responsibility.
- It's convenient that he can find something to blame.
- Come on. Get over it.
- Does he really think all that navel gazing is going to help?

As I mentioned earlier, it was a liberating and break-through moment when, in a counseling session, my therapist leaned forward, looked me in the eyes, assured me that I had experienced trauma and, more importantly, encouraged me to stop comparing myself to others and to get the help I needed in order to start working through it.

I do not like to think of myself as weak. I played rugby for 25 years, was concussed many times, broke 9 bones, and was stitched up multiple times. I was in 2 separate roll-over car accidents. I ski, snow-board, cycle and climb mountains. I've hiked the rugged 75 km West Coast Trail 3 times. I've jumped out of a plane and hang-glided.

This willingness to take risks, my thick-headed bravado and outright stupidity, is contrasted by a fear of failure, a fragile ego, and an unhealthy need to appear like I have my shit together.

I have to work bloody hard to ignore the real or imagined skeptics. However, there is a balance between on one hand admitting that we have trauma and embracing the work, and on the other extreme becoming trapped in self-pity and a victim mentality. As a woman shared in a support group I attended, "the only thing you'll get from sitting on the pity pot is a red ring around your ass!"

Gabor Maté exhorts us to avoid blame shifting and the nauseously unattractive victim mentality:

"...not getting caught in a never-ending vortex of pain, melancholy and especially victimhood. A new and rigid identity founded on "trauma" or for that matter "healing" can be its own kind of trap."
– Gabor Maté, *The Myth of Normal*

I am grateful for Gabor Maté's willingness to be vulnerable. In The Myth of Normal he recounts the story of what could seem like an immature reaction to his wife not meeting him at the airport for a scheduled pick up after a long flight. He is self-aware enough to join the dots and connect his emotions and reactions as a 70-something year-old to the trauma of his childhood where he, his mother and family suffered greatly under the Nazi's.

His wife, who obviously knows his back story and how it mani-fests in their marriage was able to lovingly but directly call him on his behavior and tell him, "come on - you can't blame Hitler for everything".

In another part of the same book, I am again endeared to Maté as he exposes himself, this time at the hands of his friend, colleague, and fellow world-renowned trauma specialist, Bessel van der Kolk.

During a conversation over lunch, van der Kolk says to Maté, "you can't drag Auschwitz around forever, Gabor."

I admire that Maté and van der Kolk have a close enough relationship that such a comment is helpful and appropriate. What a refreshing insight this was into a friendship between world-renowned researchers/authors/pioneers, and what a helpful model for the rest of us. They have not placed themselves on pedestals of self-importance, arrogance and academic theory, but are living their teachings out, and are willing to share real-life, across-the-lunch-table companionship.

Following the examples they set, when we address our own trauma, we have to remember that it is unhelpful to wallow in self-pity or otherwise become all-consumed by the trauma itself.

"This is the true joy in life, the being used for a purpose recognized by yourself as a mighty one, the being a force of nature, instead of a feverish, selfish little clod of ailments and grievances complaining that the world will not devote itself to make you happy."
– George Bernard Shaw

PART TWO
NOW YOU TELL ME?!
AKA: STUFF I WISH I KNEW BEFORE I STARTED TRAUMA THERAPY

CHAPTER 8
DON'T WORRY, IT WILL GET WORSE

Well it looks like the road to heaven
But it feels like the road to hell
— George Michael: "Freedom! '90"

It will get worse before it gets better (but it will get better).

I wish I had known a few years ago when I started my trauma healing journey that my symptoms would get worse before they got better. While this principle is mentioned in passing in the literature, stories and discussions around trauma therapy, it is grossly understated and so subtle that it is almost hidden. Yet it is such a vital concept to be aware of.

I assumed that when my trauma therapists told me to try somatics and psychedelics they were directing me towards modalities that would immediately bring relief and transformation. As I looked into it, I was encouraged by the stories and accounts of those who had benefited from these therapies.

When I eventually began experimenting with various forms of somatic therapy I often felt better for hours and even days after therapy sessions and medicine events. But at other times my symptoms would flare up almost immediately. Either way, my symptoms seemed to return. At times it felt like I was making slow progress, but most often it seemed that I was standing still or regressing.

Fortunately I had a stubborn intuition to keep going. Like a Viking sailing into the unknown in rough seas, I was driven by a hope that a *strange new land* would appear, a term I would discover a year into my journey in Peter Levine's book, *Waking the Tiger*.

It wasn't until this book was nearing completion that I came across a video, "EMDR: 3 Things I Wish I'd Known Before I Started Trauma Therapy"[1], by Dr. Pooky Knightsmith. I love Pooky for a number of reasons:

- Her name; Pooky.
- Dr. Pooky really knows her stuff and delivers solid material but in a down-to-earth informal way that I find comforting and endearing.
- She steps off screen to grab her coffee mid-video.
- The three things from her YouTube video that she wishes she had known before starting trauma therapy;

1. It would get worse before it gets better
2. It works
3. You don't have to talk about everything

are three of the things that had already prompted me to write this book.

I knew I was on the right path when I realized I was singing from the same song sheet as an expert like Pooky.

I agree with Dr. Pooky's opinion in which she candidly and with emphasis states:

"I wish I had known and had a full appreciation of the fact that it was going to get worse, before it got better. No like, worse, worse, worse ... really worse - before it got better."

Although she is referring specifically to her experience with EMDR, (a form of therapy involving eye movement that will be discussed later in Part 4, this principle of things getting worse applies across the spectrum of trauma therapies, not just EMDR).

I should note that for some people it may not actually get worse. I am pessimistically exaggerating. The dramatic provocation is intentional. My goal is not to scare anyone away from somatics but actually the complete opposite. I hope to attract people to the modalities I discuss and to instill perseverance and hope. I am hoping that having our eyes wide open from the beginning will inspire us to carry on through a predictable and necessary phase where there is little progress, or even regression.

MAYBE IT ONLY LOOKS LIKE IT'S GETTING WORSE

In reality it may only be our perception that things are getting worse. If we carry the expectation of short-term relief or a quick fix, and we don't find it, the status quo continuation of our symptoms can be perceived as worsening. Before we sought healing we probably developed an acceptance or degree of tolerance to our pain. Now, as we seek to resolve it and step into self-awareness and emotional intelligence, we become acutely aware of it. It may be that it only feels like it is getting worse.

In the video "A Simple Exercise to Ease Despair with Peter Levine, PhD" | *NICABM*[2], Levine offers a warning that even a simple exercise intended to ease despair can activate unpleasant symptoms:

"...know that it can bring up certain feelings and emotions, and of course sensations that may have been there for a long time but not acknowledged."

Levine's words of caution, and especially the simple explanation that follows, are very helpful.

Before I learned that things may initially get worse, I could not understand why some somatic exercises resulted in the return of undesirable symptoms. Often I would experience a short-lived sense of release or catharsis during a somatic exercise, but the re-emergence of issues that had been long-buried and unacknowledged would cause discomfort or re-triggering phenomenon.

YOGA TERROR

I almost fell off my chair while watching the YouTube video "Bessell van der Kolk: Overcome Trauma With Yoga"[3], in which the main point he is trying to make is that yoga is really good for treating trauma.

When discussing the benefits of yoga, van der Kolk explains how research indicates that regularly practising yoga is more effective for a traumatized person than any studied medication. So far so good. Every somatic counsellor, massage therapist, physio and hands-on practitioner I worked with told me that yoga was good for trauma and I should do it.

I eventually bought a membership at the local yoga studio. I made a practice of going regularly for months and doing my best to twist and stretch my old stiff frame in acquiescence to the young willowy instructors. I was enjoying the classes and feeling more flexible and fit, but my mental and emotional symptoms were still on a roller coaster - I didn't feel the yoga was helping.

It was the next part of van der Kolk's elucidation in the video that was a shocking but comforting revelation:

"But that doesn't mean that yoga is going to immediately make you feel better. What we find, actually, is that with people who start doing yoga, starting to feel your body may bring up feelings of helplessness, terror, etcetera, etcetera [emphasis added]."

What the ...?!! Are you kidding me?!

I couldn't believe that no one had told me that instead of making me feel better, yoga could make me feel "helpless, terrified etcetera, etcetera." It may have been at this moment that I decided to write a book. Someone needed to say the quiet part out loud and amplify this understated truth.

This was good news! I was so encouraged. My symptoms had not subsided, but now I had hope that perhaps I was making progress.

What van der Kolk said is exactly what was happening for me: feelings of helplessness, terror, and a huge amount of etcetera, etcetera!

BLESSINGS FROM BESSEL

It was a short time later while reading *The Body Keeps the Score*, that I came across a story that was eerily and wildly relevant for me.

But before I relay the story from van der Kolk's book, I have to share my own backstory:

I was at a hot yoga class and the instructor had directed us to do the Happy Baby Pose. As I mention later in the book, I am only learning to be aware of the Felt Sense, and what my body is communicating to my mind. While holding this pose - awkwardly and with difficulty - I had a hazy inner perception of myself as a frightened infant. At the time I had no idea whether it was something oddly real or my imagination. It soon dropped from my conscience as we moved on to other poses.

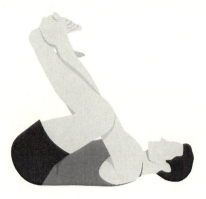

I don't know what my feelings or emotions were after the class. But I do know that after months of purposefully abstaining from alcohol, I went straight to the liquor store.

It wasn't until a few days later that the thought occurred to me: "I wonder if that Happy Baby Pose and my sense of fear had anything to do with me suddenly wanting to drink the other night?"

This is when I came across the eerily relevant account in *The Body Keeps the Score*. In it, van der Kolk summarizes his time with a patient, whom he calls "Annie" for the sake of the story. Annie had been a rape victim, and she was having trouble with some poses from her yoga therapy. The one pose that was the hardest was Happy Baby.

Now, my trauma is quite different from Annie's; it is easy to see why the position of Happy Baby would be triggering for her. But it was the last line that jumped out for me and provided immense comfort, relief and assurance that I was on the right path:

"Learning how to comfortably assume Happy Baby is a challenge for many patients in our yoga classes."
**– Bessel van der Kolk, *The Body Keeps the Score*
(pg. 274)**

I was not alone! I almost started to cry when I read the story. No wonder my symptoms flared up during yoga. No wonder that I went from Cheerful Baby to Fearful Baby to Beer-ful Baby.

I was getting better. Even though, that night, it felt like things were getting worse.

I am happy to share that as I continued my yoga practice and Happy Baby Pose my symptoms progressively became less problematic. And the Felt Sense and imagery I was experiencing changed over the following months. The extreme fear began to lessen, then in later sessions joy came, then deep laughter.

One time, while in the pose, I had a profound sense of attunement with my mother, then my father - a loving, calm, eye to eye, soul to soul gaze. Authentic child and parent connection as it was meant to be. It felt so healing - and I believe it was.

As their titles suggest, the following two videos provide additional explanation about why things may get worse when we begin somatic practices:

"How Meditation May Make Nervous System Dysregulation Worse" - Jessica Maguire[4]

"Why We Can Get Overwhelmed When We Start Healing Our Trauma" - Irene Lyon[5]

Here are a few questions posted by Redditors who experienced things getting worse after they began somatics:
From r/SomaticExperiencing:

 People often say, "It gets worse before it gets better." For those further along, has that been your experience and how did you manage it with SE?

...I have blocked such big things for so long and many folks say, "it gets worse before it gets better". I accept some aspects of that but it's such a hard thing to swallow.

Too much too quickly?

I had my first IFS session virtually yesterday and it led to one of the worst panic attacks I've had in a while...

 Since starting somatic work do you feel more afraid/confused as your system is reopening from freeze/blocked feelings?

So although, when you first start working through your trauma, it may seem to get worse—keep going! I know it may be difficult, but I encourage you to persevere. The therapists, experts and practitioners agree - things will get better: eventually. We just need to keep going.

CHAPTER 9
RELAPSE

There is no shame in relapse.

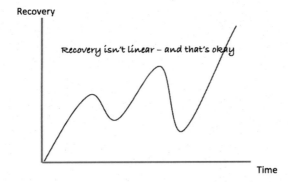

When I use the word relapse I am referring to a recurrence of one or more of the many symptoms of trauma. This is not an exhaustive list:

- anger
- fear

- sadness
- shame
- confusion
- anxiety[1]
- depression[2]
- numbness
- guilt
- hopelessness
- irritability
- difficulty concentrating
- headaches[3]
- digestive symptoms
- fatigue[4]
- racing heart
- sweating
- feeling jumpy
- substance use
- suicidal thoughts

Relapse is not only a descriptor for substance use or a return to undesired alcohol or drug use. I understand the seriousness and life and death implications of that form of relapse. I am not minimizing or trivializing its unique elements. However, I am grouping it together with other symptoms of trauma in order to:

- Discuss it as a surface manifestation of an underlying cause
- Identify it as one symptom amongst many other symptoms
- Remove the shame and stigma associated with addiction
- Remove the added guilt and sense of failure that drug and alcohol users carry
- Focus attention and healing on the underlying pain

- Level the symptomatic field so that some sufferers don't feel worse or better, compared to others
- Remove the moralizing, grading, or blaming associated with some symptoms

Stigma and shame around relapse related to substance use cause sufferers to hide, isolate and often use alone. My province's top doctor, Dr. Bonnie Henry perceptively stated during a discussion regarding B.C.'s overdose death epidemic; "these sufferers are stuck in a cycle of chronic relapse."

While substance use and abuse in themselves carry their own bundle of stigmatizing stereotypes and debilitating perceptions, being a "relapser" adds additional weight and crippling, sometimes fatal burdens. It is my belief that there are three general groupings of substance/alcohol users:

1. Those who are not currently drinking/using; abstinent, sober, "in recovery".
2. Those who are actively and intentionally drinking or using; not seeking recovery, utilizing harm reduction, safe supply etc.
3. A middle group who want to drink or use less (abstinence or not), and have attempted to control or stop their drinking/using but are stuck in a cycle of undesired recurrence.

THEY WALK AMONGST US

I suggest that it is this third group that is the largest and most invisible; suffering deeply and often alone, and as Dr. Bonnie suggests, dying. I believe more compassion and attention should be provided for this group of often very functional people within our communities. One of my goals is to illuminate this issue and help find solutions.

As we address our trauma, a retriggering session or intense retraumatization may bring about a recurrence of one or more symptoms. We may freeze, we may have an anxiety attack, we may experience a shit-storm in our brain, or we may compulsively numb the pain with alcohol or other drugs. Piling on guilt, shame and attributing a monstrous sense of failure to one symptom in comparison to another is illogical, unhelpful, and often fatal.

MAYBE YOU WON'T RELAPSE

It is my hope and prayer that recurrences of symptoms don't occur, but the reality is that they may. We may not see radical improvement in the short term - things may stay the same, or even feel worse - but they will get better.

When those shitty times hit you, it is normal for you to experience a relapse of your symptoms. Maybe you won't, but if you do, try not to feel worse about some symptoms in comparison to others.

CHAPTER 10
WHY IS THIS TAKING ... SO ... BLOODY ... LONG?

When I awoke today, suddenly nothing happened
But in my dreams, I slew the dragon
And down this beaten path, up this cobbled lane
I'm walking in my old footsteps, once again
– Colin Hay: "Waiting for My Real Life to Begin"[1]

T ypically when we injure ourselves or are diagnosed with a physical condition requiring medical care we ask our doctor the question, "How long until I'm better?" Quite often there are well-established timeframes for rehabilitation, and we can plan our lives with some certainty or at least probabilities.

Sorry, healing from trauma is not like that.

How long will it take? is a common question from Redditors. I'd recommend checking out some content from r/SomaticExperiencing, such as:

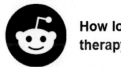 **How long did it take for somatic experiencing therapy to change your life?**

How long did it take for SE to start "working" for you? i.e. How long before you noticed small/bigger changes?

 How long have you been doing somatic experiencing for?

 How long into somatic therapy did you start to experience significant positive changes?

 How long before you started feeling some improvement?

I haven't found any research or references that speak specifically about what to expect as far as timeframes for noticcable relief from symptoms. Many of the accounts in Maté's, van der Kolk's and Levine's books mention moments of relief in therapy sessions, but many others indicate that longer periods of time are the norm before a significant breakthrough.

In the video, "[Trauma Tip #6] How Long Does It Take to Heal Trauma?"[2], Irene Lyons offers some great insights. She suggests shifting the script behind the "how long does it take?" question.

"There needs to be this different perspective that sees this world of healing the nervous system as lifestyle and life-long. ... There's never-ending elements to feel, and revise, and notice and uncover."

In our fast paced world of project plans, agendas and promises of quick fixes, the lack of identifiable milestones and a finish line may be frustrating.

I asked a trauma therapist for an idea of when I could expect to see improvement if I stuck to the program. He provided a rough, "no promises", timeline with markers at 30 days, 90 days, 9 months and two years.

30 Days - Look for some kind of indication that a shift is beginning, or a short period of improvement. It might be only a few moments of relief during a session or practice. A glimpse or a whisper.

90 Days - A clearer sense that you are making progress. Some symptoms are less severe, others may still be problematic.

9 Months - Significant breakthroughs. Things are not perfect but you notice some serious progression. Keep going.

2 Years - Don't be surprised that your life is getting better. You deserve that.

This loose framework kept me motivated and was fairly accurate. Mind you, I was quite aggressive, was able to devote a significant amount of time and effort, and was fairly disciplined in maintaining a regular routine. As I mention in my later discussion of Macro-pendulation, sometimes being aggressive means taking days off, or multiple days off, lots of rest, and lots of self-care.

When Gabor Maté was asked in the interview "Gabor Maté on Psychedelics, Trauma and the Body (Part 5)"[3] "can trauma ever be fully healed?", his response includes him humorously sharing his desire that the epitaph he wants on his gravestone is, "It was a lot more work than I had anticipated."

I have a couple of friends my age who are working through significant transformation, and still waiting for more. I remind them that we are in the KFC program. Colonel Sanders didn't start KFC until he was 65. We still have a few years to discover the 11 herbs and spices for our secret recipe.

In our society, we expect quick results. However, we have to give ourselves time for the answers to come, the injuries to heal, and the growth and transformation to put down roots.

> *"It's gonna happen soon, soon, oh, so very soon*
> *It's just that times are lean*
> *And you say, be still my love*
> *Open up your heart, let the light shine in*
> *Don't you understand*
> *Oh, I already have a plan"*
> **Colin Hay: "Waiting for My Real Life to Begin"**[4]

CHAPTER 11
TOOLS TO MINIMIZE RETRAUMATIZATION

As I have mentioned, when I began to explore the world of somatic practice, I found the warnings about *things getting worse* to be understated. In fact they were so obscure I didn't even notice them. To counter that obscurity I have overstated this warning and exaggerated the probability that things will get worse. It is not a certainty.

A trained trauma therapist should be able to provide guidance that prevents or minimizes retraumatization or an increased occurrence of symptoms. The problem for me was that there are few trauma therapists and they are often booking months down the road. I was unwilling to wait for professional help. I learned to apply the following principles on my own.

SLOWER IS BETTER

I find it very hard to be patient and go slow. If someone tells me that an exercise is good for me, I want to do it as intensely and as often as possible. Pendulation and titration are two practices that have been developed to slow trauma therapy down to a pace that is of maximum benefit.

PENDULATION

This term was coined by Peter Levine and demonstrated by him in the video, "What is Pendulation in Somatic Experiencing® with Peter A Levine, PhD"[1]. Essentially, like a pendulum, the concept is to sway back and forth between emotions and sensations of contraction and expansion: an ebb and a flow, if you will. Gradually, the two polar states become integrated:

> *"It is the holding together of these polarities that facilitates deep integration and often an 'alchemical' transformation."*

TITRATION

Titration is a word borrowed from chemistry in which chemicals are added or mixed in very small amounts in order to measure and monitor the desired response or chemical reaction. The aim of somatic titration is to slow trauma work down to avoid overload by conducting therapy in small amounts. Therapy or practices occur in very small doses with ample pauses for processing, integration and adjustment. The person is only exposed to as much work as they can handle in a particular practice.

MACRO-PENDULATION

This is a term I coined to describe a personal practice I have developed. As previously discussed, all the experts strongly advise that somatic therapy be conducted slowly (slower is faster) and to use titration and pendulation.

However, sometimes I overdo it and my system gets completely out of balance or dysregulated. This can be a dangerous place for me to be, with symptoms manifesting to an extreme. At these times I have started to practice macro-pendulation.

Levine's pendulation, as described earlier, is applied when a therapist pulls a client in and out of activation or stimulation during therapy sessions by using periods of pause and relaxation. Pendulation of this variety is conducted on a scale of minutes in and out of intensity - what I call micro-pendulation.

Macro-pendulation is conducted over hours or days. When an intense period of therapy, or somatic experiencing or active healing takes place, I find it absolutely necessary to fully disengage from the process.

Often after a positive event or treatment session, I need to take time for restabilization and adjustment. I may feel energized and even euphoric. This is not the time to pile on more somatics, complete a to-do list, or save the world - even though I may feel like it. In this moment, I need to be intentional and:

- Relax
- Rest
- Practice self-care
- Reflect
- Walk
- Gaze
- Get in nature
- Spend time alone, or with a safe, intimate person.
- Call a good friend and share what I'm going through

I'll give three examples of when I have practiced macro-pendulation:

COACHING OVERLOAD

I had a Somatic Coach who came into my life at a point when I was floundering and looking for solutions. He was divinely deposited in my path just when I needed him. He has a unique approach that met my needs in a providential way. His compassion, understanding and encouragement was remarkable and healing in itself.

One element of his approach that most therapists seem to disagree with is to work repetitively and intensely rather than slowly or with titration and pendulation. In addition to our weekly one hour sessions he would advise me to do multiple sessions each day.

At this time, I was also exploring breathwork, cold immersion, sauna, massage, EMDR, vagus nerve activation, hot yoga, talk therapy, sound baths etc. and many other techniques. Basically whatever I came across I tried. He encouraged me to do multiple sessions each day involving a number of activities. And I believe it worked, eventually. Even though I would have recurrences of a variety of symptoms, I had a clear sense that I was moving forward. But I had to learn to take days or even a week off to recover.

JFMSU

As I mentioned above, I learned as many somatic techniques as I could in a very short period of time. I began to do a number of them back-to-back or even multiple practices at the same time (This was in the first few months of my exploration and experimentation with somatics - I do not recommend this).

For instance I would have a sauna, do 5 minutes of Wim Hoff breathing, then stand in the freezing-cold ocean up to my neck while doing EMDR, sunlight therapy, vagus nerve ear massage, and breathwork, alternating with self-compassion affirmations. Then sometimes I would return inside to do a sound bath with drumming, tuning fork and singing bowl, then finish with self-massage, more vagus nerve exercises, Voo sound, EMDR and sphincter contractions. Yup, craziness. I am not recommending it.

I heard that this method of doing multiple somatics back to back, or all at once, is referred to as layering. I called it stacking, but later labelled this overloading technique JFMSU - Just F*** My Shit Up.

I sure needed macro-pendulation after those sessions. Eventually I began to heed the majority voice of the somatic therapy community and pulled the throttle way back. Now, I go a lot slower, titrate and micro-pendulate, as well as macro-pendulate. Occasionally I will stack 2 or 3 techniques, but only for a short period of time.

UNINTENDED THERAPY

I use this term to describe those times when I have encountered a transformational moment or healing event completely out of the blue. One time I had an unexpected conversation with a respected medical doctor regarding psychedelics and mental health. It was very encouraging and enlightening and provided me with confirmation that I was on the right path. I was pumped with energy and had difficulty getting to sleep.

The next day I was giddy and manic. The previous evening had been overwhelmingly positive, but I was in a worse place mentally, emotionally and somatically than I was before my conversation with the doctor. I had made a leap forward in my healing journey, but was temporarily going backwards in my emotional and nervous system regulation.

Fortunately, by this time I was starting to gain some self-awareness and realized I needed to practice macro-pendulation. Rest, relax, and integrate. So I did. I went for a walk beside the ocean. I napped. I had a sauna. I phoned a friend. I watched some Netflix.

SOMATIC KINDERGARTEN

I made mistakes in my early days of somatic experimentation. Fortunately the recurrences of my symptoms and "things getting worse before they got better", did not carry more severe consequences. I suppose I will never know if it would have been more effective to move radically more slowly, as the experts suggest. I suppose it would have been safer, at least to some degree.

Regardless, I continue to practice macro-pendulation when either out of ignorance, bull-ish stupidity, or in response to instruction or guidance, I over do it.

If you find that you sometimes overdue your somatics, taking time to recover from intensive periods of therapy may be an essential part of your healing journey. Slower is better, titration, micro-pendulation and macro-pendulation are essentials for the somatic toolbox.

CHAPTER 12
YOU DON'T HAVE TO TALK ABOUT IT

"Therapists have an undying faith in the capacity of talk to resolve trauma."
— Bessel van der Kolk, *The Body Keeps the Score* (pg. 233)

Historically, talk therapy has been the main modality for healing trauma. In the chapter, Language: Miracle and Tyranny of *The Body Keeps the Score*, van der Kolk wonderfully details both the benefits and drawbacks involved in putting our stories into words.

Most specialists strongly recommend talking about our trauma and I fully agree. Once again, my objective is to make trauma and somatic therapy as accessible and inviting as possible. To illuminate hidden or underutilized entry points into healing for others who:

- can't recall their trauma
- are unable to talk about it
- are unwilling to talk about it, either consciously or subconsciously

- don't want to talk about it
- can't put it into words
- have talked about it extensively and exhausted that modality

A plethora of resources on talk therapy are available, but the information on non-talk trauma therapy is comparatively scant. Even most somatic or body-based therapies require the client to talk about their trauma to some degree. Some trauma sufferers may be relieved to receive permission to "not talk."

After years of talk therapy, I became disillusioned about the benefits of recounting my limited and unclear understanding of my past to yet another therapist. It didn't really seem to be helping. Or perhaps it helped early on, but the benefits of talk had been realized and maximized years ago - I needed some additional tools for deeper excavation.

Our recollection of trauma can take a number of forms:

1. Specific - an event, words, an accident, physical abuse, sexual assault
2. Prolonged - systemic racism, chronic fear of a parent, sustained terror, psychological abuse
3. *Second hand or shared - accounts and stories from others aware of your experience
4. *Reasonable conclusions - specific accounts are not available, but connecting the dots points to traumatic events or situations.
5. *Hunches, dreams and intuitive knowledge (see the video "Cultivating Transgenerational Resilience: Healing Ancestral Trauma"[1] - near the beginning and then around 25 mins.)
6. *No recollection - the person has no information or recollection, but the symptoms of trauma are apparent.

7. Terror and the terrible - some traumatic events are almost impossible to put into words.

* Especially relevant to early childhood, infancy, pre-birth, and transgenerational trauma

While talk therapy has been the main modality for healing trauma, in the case of 6 above, it is impossible to describe one's unrecalled trauma. Trauma in 7 is locked away and too terrifying to verbalize. Furthermore, trauma falling into categories 3, 4, and 5 may be quite fuzzy and difficult to express. Significant guidance and assistance may be required to put some traumatizing situations into words, or to feel safe enough to do so.

Don't just take my word for it. You can find plenty of Redditors and other online community members describing their challenges in identifying their trauma. Two that resonated with me were:

I read about Somatic Experiencing recently. Would it be useful when you are not sure of what exactly is the trauma you had faced, but something you have accumulated little by little over years, and is now impeding your daily life? Secondly, can someone self practice the same using any exercises?

What are peoples' experiences using Somatic Experiencing for preverbal or even in womb trauma?

A recent article in *Hindustan Times* titled "Key Signs of Childhood Emotional Neglect" outlines that:

1. Sustained or prolonged emotional and relational trauma can be just as harmful as an event-based trauma such as an accident, abuse or assault.

2. It is often difficult, and perhaps even impossible to clearly identify early traumatic experiences because it occurred in infancy or early childhood, and there was no aberration from a well-established and clearly identifiable norm. How could a child, or an adult looking back, objectively say, "well xyz is what happened to me, but abc is what should have happened"?

"However, because it's not easy to pinpoint when and where the emotional wounds occurred, it can be challenging to recognise and overcome them."
– Therapist Emmylou Antonieth Seaman

Although most of the stories and case studies that trauma specialists write about appear to involve talking or dialogue, I was both relieved and amused by van der Kolk's account of an EMDR session where the individual wanted help with a painful childhood trauma, but didn't want to discuss the specific incidents. This was new to van der Kolk, who described himself as "annoyed and flustered."

After the session the individual reported that the matter of his trauma had been resolved, but van der Kolk was skeptical and concluded that without his patient sharing what had occurred during their session, he would be unable to say for sure whether it was truly resolved.

In the end, van der Kolk shares that he continues to be fascinated with the issue that it may be possible for people to heal without talking about their trauma.

Although this particular account was relative to an EMDR session, my uneducated guess is that it is not the only somatic modality friendly to a non-talk approach.

Not having to talk about trauma may be a relief and comfort to some, and could provide an entry point into a long-needed healing journey and away from a crippling past. To be sure, becoming aware, confronting and talking about one's history and trauma is essential in most cases, I simply hope to facilitate the consideration of an opportunity for healing that has been understated or ignored - and which may lead to a breakthrough for some.

In the YouTube video, "Telling Your Story Just Might Be Retraumatizing You"[2], therapist Anna Runkle, who labels herself "The Crappy Childhood Fairy" (*love it*), provides some insights into why talking...and talking...and talking... about our trauma can make us feel worse and may prevent us from moving forward in our healing.

Talking about my trauma, dialoguing, and getting feedback from specialists was essential for me. But in some cases, or at some point, something more than talk, or less talk, or no talk is what was needed.

HOW DO WE TALK ABOUT SOMETHING WE CAN'T RECALL?

Psychiatrist Thomas Verny theorizes that although we may not be able to consciously remember our intrauterine experiences, these memories do still exist subconsciously, accessible as emotional imprints, recorded in our body cells. He calls this process "bodywide memory."

Peter Levine provides comforting assurance that even if we can't remember our trauma, we can resolve our symptoms:

"You have not been irreversibly damaged, and it is possible to diminish or even eliminate your symptoms."
– Peter Levine, *Waking the Tiger* (pg. 5)

DR. POOKIE!

As mentioned, I really like the way Dr. Pookie Knightsmith communicates serious and complex issues in a simple and down to earth style. In her YouTube video "EMDR: 3 Things I Wish I'd Known Before I Started Trauma Therapy"[3] she talks about how even though she trusted her therapist and had a long history with him, she was terrified to talk about certain things. She was relieved to find out she didn't have to talk about anything she didn't want to and in fact spent most of her sessions silent.

TENSION AND TRAUMA RELEASING EXERCISES (TRE)

Some practices specifically provide for the avoidance of talk therapy. TRE is a somatic technique developed by Dr. David Berceli and described in this video, "TRE: A Condensed Explanation."[4] TRE is a body based process which can allow the individual to discharge tension from the body, and does not require "revisiting the story" (ie: verbally describing or talking about the traumatic experience).

So as you can see, although talk therapy is valuable, you can get on your healing path without it—you may even travel most of your way down that path without it, and that's okay!

CHAPTER 13
WELCOME TO AA

But I can't feel anything.

H i, my name is Hans and I'm an alexithymiac.
       I was so glad to find out I had alexithymia. I have since met others with this condition and we jokingly, or maybe not, talk about starting a self-help group called Alexithymiacs Anonymous.

"Alexithymia, also known as emotional blindness, is a personality feature in which a person has difficulty experiencing, identifying, understanding, and expressing their emotions."
– Psychology Today[1]

Alexithymia manifested for me in two ways. First, I have always found it difficult to identify and describe my feelings. The best I could often do was to describe my feelings as "a shit storm in my head."

Second, as I began to receive somatic therapy, I found it impossible to identify any sensations or areas in my body where my trauma was situated or manifesting.

Typically, somatic therapists will ask questions like:

- When you describe your trauma, what do you feel in your body?
- What area in your body carries your trauma?
- Where in your body do you feel stress?
- Does stress or tension move to other parts of your body?
- If I ask you to take a few deep breaths, can you describe what you feel within your body?
- Can you describe what you are feeling in your body at this moment?
- Based on what you are feeling, do you have an idea of what you need today?

Those questions frustrated me. I did not have a clue how to answer. After years of resisting trauma work and then now finally doing it, it was disconcerting to be informed that trauma resided in my body, and that I needed to gain some sense of where and how my trauma manifested physically.

"In order to overcome trauma, you need help to get back in touch with your body, with your Self."
– Bessel van der Kolk, The Body Keeps the Score (pg. 249)

I found my first few sessions of somatic therapy difficult. My therapist had me talk about specific traumatic events for a few minutes. Then she would ask what physical sensations I was feeling, and whether I could identify where the locked up traumatic energy was situated in my body.

I felt the need to come up with something. I thought to myself, "well my glasses are kind of bugging the bridge of my nose; and I felt some indigestion from the spicy burrito I had for lunch; also my underwear were kind of tight." (It was a bad laundry day where I had to wear that pair of underwear from the back of the drawer. You know, the ones that are too small, but you keep them because they are still perfectly good - they are the only option when everything else is the laundry bin.)

Too much information? Anyways, I had nothing to report to my therapist as far as bodily connection to my feelings, emotions or trauma. And I was trying, I really was! She assured me that this was normal for someone addressing trauma for the first time and encouraged me to be patient and kind to myself.

My desire to get in touch with my body and feelings increased when I read Peter Levine's lengthy chapter on "The Felt Sense" in his book, *Waking the Tiger*. His complex description of the "Felt Sense," or internal body sensations, and his explanation of their useful benefits, was on one hand compelling and inviting, but on the other seemingly unattainable for me:

"In directing our attention to these internal body sensations, rather than attacking the trauma head-on, we can unbind and free the energies that have been in check."
– Peter Levine, *Waking the Tiger*

This supposed freedom and unbinding sounds great, Peter, but I can't feel anything!

Significant comfort and relief came through Bessel van der Kolk's book, *The Body Keeps the Score*, where he explains that traumatized people often have trouble sensing what is going on in their bodies. Because of this, they often can't tell what, precisely, is upsetting them.

But take heart, we can get better:

"People with alexithymia can get better only by learning to recognize the relationship between their physical sensations and their emotions, much as colorblind people can only enter the world of color by learning to distinguish and appreciate shades of gray."

– **Bessel van der Kolk,** *The Body Keeps the Score*
(**pg. 101**)

This describes my experience. While I used to find it so frustrating to identify what I was feeling, and also correlate my feelings to any sensation in my body, I am now beginning to identify shades of gray.

REVERSE ENGINEERING THE FELT SENSE AND SOMATIC HEALING

In an effort to heal from alexithymia and develop my Felt Sense, I decided to apply the basic principles of reverse engineering. By this I mean, if I couldn't identify what was happening in my body after becoming aware of a feeling, how about if I reversed the process and first focused on an area of my body, and then sought to become aware of any feelings and emotions related to my trauma that were connected to that area?

I needed to get someone physically touching me or working on my body. I proceeded to book at least one massage appointment per week with a variety of massage practitioners. I would ask them to work deeply with significant pressure. As they began the massage, I would tell them that I was doing somatic counseling and trauma informed therapy. I asked them if it was okay if I talked about whatever came to mind as they worked on different parts of my body, and also invited them to give me feedback or input. They were quick to remind me that they were not counselors, psychologists or mental health therapists.

Some remained very quiet during the treatment and refrained from dialogue. Others, and these were the ones I returned to, gave me helpful "off the record" informal feedback, and valuable input. Over a few months those sessions helped me to become aware of mind-body connections, and correlate bodily sensations to emotions and feelings.

This process may sound forced, mechanical or primitive, but it was a good start for me.

To find what may work for you, search for what may have worked for others. Like me, perhaps you can relate to this Redditor:

 How to feel your feelings?

How do you know if you're truly feeling your feelings? I'm doing talk therapy and somatic body work on my own at home. If you don't have a point of reference, how do you truly know if you are feeling your emotions? Or if you're just fooling yourself into thinking you are?

By seeing what worked for them, you can learn to develop your own Felt Sense; you don't need to be able to instinctively connect your feelings and emotions to your trauma in order to work through it. We can gradually learn to see shades of gray, and perhaps, eventually, vivid colors.

PART THREE
TIPS FOR THE JOURNEY

1. You Are Your Guide

2. Try Everything/Multiple Pathways

3. Self-Compassion

CHAPTER 14
YOU ARE YOUR GUIDE

Lights will guide you home
And ignite your bones
– Coldplay: "Fix You"

"No one can plot somebody else's course of healing, because that's not how healing works. There are no road maps for something that must find its own individual arc."
– Gabor Maté, *The Myth of Normal* (pg. 374)

"Our bodies (instincts) will tell us where the blockages are and when we are moving too fast. Our intellects can tell us how to regulate the experience so that we are not overwhelmed."
– Peter Levine, *Waking the Tiger* (pg. 18)

"The exercise of agency is powerfully healing."
– Gabor Maté, *The Myth of Normal* (pg. 377)

P rofessional therapists, medical practitioners and science-based experts are essential. They are my fundamental source of guidance. In my journey to heal from trauma I have benefited from the first-hand advice of medical doctors, mental health and addiction psychologists, professional counselors, massage therapists, physiotherapists and chiropractors. I am confidently reliant on their education, training, experience and the oversight of their professional colleges and governing bodies.

Further to this, I rely fully on evidence-based practices, peer-reviewed research, and proven approaches to healing. The surge in criticism of proven medical practices and the flocking towards independent approaches in regards to recent global health issues is troubling and puzzling to me. But don't get me going.

While relying on the underlying and over-arching guidance of medical and health professionals, I have found it beneficial to take on some responsibility and agency as I sought to heal from trauma. It is possible to practice a healthy degree of independence and autonomy, without becoming wildly rebellious, independent, or latching on to conspiracy theories and fear-based silliness.

When I decided to get serious about addressing my trauma I was unable to find the help of a trained trauma informed somatic therapist in my area who had any available openings. Therefore I began to read and research somatic tools and techniques and experimented on my own. Although it was a roller coaster ride with occasional recurrences of a variety of symptoms I was encouraged by Peter Levine's remarks in his prologue to *Waking the Tiger*:

"If you are in therapy, it may be helpful to share this book with your therapist. If you are not in therapy, it is possible to use this book to help yourself."
– Peter Levine, *Waking the Tiger*

It was liberating to find out that if professional guidance from others wasn't available it was okay to help myself. This permitted me to experiment, be creative, and tap into my body-mind intuition. As Maté says, "there are no road maps", so I had to, in part, make my own road. I found it to be an exhilarating adventure with twists, wrong turns, and the odd crash into the ditch, but one that led to some amazing experiences of transformation.

There are a number of reasons why it may be necessary or helpful to explore the idea of self-guidance:

- Somatics and psychedelics are relatively new fields of research and practice. New methodologies are regularly being introduced.
- There are very few specialists who are trained in these modalities, as well as trauma. Demand far exceeds supply. Some of us cannot afford to wait for an appointment only available months down the road, or in some distant locale.
- Trauma touches all parts of our being; mind, emotions, feelings, brain, nervous system, mental health, immune system, hormones, etc. Maté refers to the tongue-twisting discipline of *psychoneuroimmunoendocrinology* required to address trauma. Apparently, these holistic practitioners are out there. I was unable to find one in my area who was equipped and available.
- There is no one person, place or source of information that is going to provide everything we need. No one else is going to sort through all the options and determine what is best for you.
- Ultimately, no one knows you better than you know yourself. (I feel like I need to restate my aversion to ego-driven or fear-based independence)
- As I mentioned elsewhere, listening for the prompts, developing your intuition, and discovering your agency may be an essential part of healing. Perhaps the journey

to wellness is as vital to your well-being as the ultimate destination.

Gabor Maté, who was a practicing medical doctor for decades, knows a thing or two about the role the patient plays in their own health and treatment plan. He encourages us to have confidence in our intuitions, participate in decisions and to be our own guide:

"Another lamentable feature of Western medical practice ... is a power hierarchy that casts physicians as the exalted experts and patients as the passive recipients of care."
– Gabor Maté, *The Myth of Normal* (pg. 74)

He summarizes that this imbalance often leaves patients without the confidence to advocate for themselves, and to all-to-readily dismiss their own feelings and input towards their own healing process.

Maté's section on agency in Chapter 26 of *The Myth of Normal* is profound. We are provided with permission to evaluate things freely and fully, and to use our gut feelings. How liberating! Yet, with it comes responsibility. He closes this part with:

"Agency is neither attitude nor affect, neither blind acceptance nor a rejection of authority."
– Gabor Maté, *The Myth of Normal*

The journey of educating oneself and learning new things can bring about hope and expectation - which in themselves can aid in healing. Two years ago I was uninformed, skeptical and even critical of these modalities. Taking the time to research, gain understanding and potentially engage with new healing modalities was therapeutic - it was therapy before the therapy.

The process of becoming informed is much more than an intellectual *ascent*. It can be a whole body *assent* if we allow it to be.

Acting with agency does not mean one has to be lonely. You are not alone. I have found myself welcomed into a warm community of fellow seekers. This is another beautiful part of the process and a source of healing in itself. You will find yourself surrounded and supported by others whose path towards healing and healthy agency intertwines with yours.

For example, discussion groups like Reddit's r/SomaticExperiencing contain the questions, stories and accounts of countless others trying to figure this out and move forward in their healing.

The following posts from Reddit are just a small snapshot representing the countless sufferers who are reaching out, asking questions and being proactive in their pursuit of healing.

 Can't stop napping during the day.

 Sensation run through my knuckles and knees— anyone else?

 What to look for in a psychologist doing somatic therapy?

Remember: even with others' advice, including those of health care professionals, you are the ultimate decider when it comes to knowing what is best for you.

CHAPTER 15
TRY EVERYTHING/MULTIPLE PATHWAYS

"Which one of these is best for any particular survivor is an empirical question. Most people I have worked with require a combination."
— **Bessel van der Kolk**

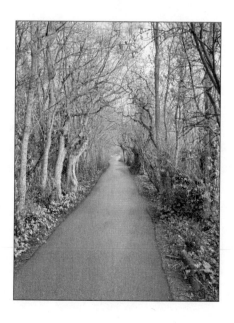

I find it interesting when someone has been helped dramatically by a certain therapy, somatic technique, recovery program or psychedelic and then becomes convinced that everyone needs it. I can understand that their evangelical fervor is caused by the amazing transformation that they have personally experienced. I am happy to celebrate with someone whose life has been changed, perhaps even saved.

But it is often not logical to assume that what worked for them will work for everyone. Bessel reminds of us this:

"I have no preferred treatment modality, as no single approach fits everybody ... Each one of them can produce profound changes, depending on the nature of the particular problem and the makeup of the individual person."
– Bessel van der Kolk, ***The Body Keeps the Score*** **(pg. 4)**

Similarly, Maté points out that each of us will have to design and navigate our personal healing journeys:

"There are no road maps for something that must find its own individual arc."
– Gabor Maté, ***The Myth of Normal*** **(pg. 374)**

Unfortunately there is no template, no easy to follow instruction manual that guarantees a completed project. There is no one sized prescription or formula that is going to work for everyone.

"What follows is not an attempt to prescribe a one-size-fits-all solution - no size does - but to point to the possibility of healing on individual and societal levels, even in the context of our increasingly anxious and disordered culture."
– Gabor Maté, ***The Myth of Normal*** **(pg. 362)**

There are numerous forms of talk therapy and a variety of medicines. The field of somatic practices is constantly broadening, along with our knowledge of underlying traumas. Bessel van der Kolk highlights 3 broad modalities of treatment:

1. Processing memories of trauma through talk and connection with the self and others
2. Restricting unwanted "alarm reactions" of the body, such as by taking medications
3. Experiencing situations and emotions that resoundingly contradict those of the trauma.

"Which one of these is best for any particular survivor is an empirical question. Most people I have worked with require a combination."
– **Bessel van der Kolk, *The Body Keeps the Score* (pg. 3)**

This closing sentence provides what I have found to be particularly good advice. Consider a combination of talk therapy, medicines and somatics.

In a YouTube interview, Bessel van der Kolk provides another helpful observation about the need to experiment and find what works best for you. He suggests that one will discover what makes them feel better by accident, by trying new things and seeing what helps. When asked why yoga is an effective tool for healing trauma he replies:

"These things are usually an issue of accident. You happen to meet someone who does yoga and that person says come do a yoga class with me, and you do that, and then you find your body feels calmer and your mind is more focused afterwards, and you say 'oh that's interesting.' ... for some people qigong may be better, or tai chi or some other musical practice. But for me yoga was a way of exploring to what degree people can change their relationship to bodily sensations."

– Bessel van der Kolk, "The 7 Surprising Ways To Heal Trauma Without Medication"[1]

As illustrated, there are multiple pathways. Explore, experiment, and eventually you'll discover the unique route that works for you.

CHAPTER 16
SELF-COMPASSION

I include self-compassion as a "tip for the journey" because it does not really fit into the somatic tools section, but definitely warrants inclusion and profile.

Self-compassion turbo-boosted my healing and as a stand-alone tool was just as powerful as psychedelics, support groups, somatics and talk therapy. Eight months ago I had never heard of it.

I have mentioned elsewhere how key messages and directions seem to serendipitously come across my path from multiple sources when the time is right. On one occasion I was scrolling through Ted Talks looking for information on trauma and somatics when I came across Dr. Kristin Neff:

"The Space Between Self-Esteem and Self Compassion" | TEDxTalks[1]

I listened for a minute or so and was mildly interested but only because what seemed to me like a fluffy insubstantial topic had made the Ted Talk stage. I moved on, looking for more meaty and relevant subject matter. Soon after, I came across a Bessel van der Kolk interview, someone I am always eager to listen to. It was a fortuitous encounter.

Van der Kolk spends the majority of this interview explaining the effectiveness of trauma treatment methods that I was already familiar with such as EMDR, mindfulness and neural feedback.

Near the end of the interview, the host asks van der Kolk if he is aware of any new and innovative techniques; what is coming in the next ten years? A portion of his response got my attention:

*"Mindfulness in and of itself has only moderate benefits, but the issue is mindfulness with **self-compassion** [emphasis added], and learning to love what you discover inside of yourself. I think meditation, love and compassion is becoming a very big issue again."*
– Bessel van der Kolk, "Bessel van der Kolk - Effective Methods for Treating Trauma"[2]

This was a "wow" moment for me. I was expecting and hoping that his thoughts on new techniques and what innovative tools are coming in the next ten years might include something like the development of an infra-red trauma sensing body scanner, or a recently discovered plant medicine from the east-facing slopes of the mountains of Uzbekistan that was fertilized by the urine of albino yaks. Not something as simplistic and accessible as self-compassion. What the heck, Bessel?!

In another video, "How the body keeps the score on trauma" | *Big Think+*[3] van der Kolk states,

"This issue of self-compassion and really knowing that your reactions are understandable and are rooted in you getting stuck in the past is a terribly important part of beginning to recover from trauma."

Really?! Self-compassion is a terribly important part of recovery? Intrigued, I went back to find Kristin Neff and her talk on self-compassion which I had passed off as fluff. For those of us who need evidence-based information and live in the world of "show me the science" and, "where's the research?" - it turns out that self-compassion is solid. Rock solid.

The research of Dr. Neff and other scholars, most of which has been done only in the last decade, proves that self-compassion can change lives. I highly recommend becoming informed on this subject and beginning a practice of self-compassion. Interestingly, Neff has found that women are less prone to practice healthy self-compassion than men.

I suggest starting with Kristin Neff's TEDx Talk[4] and website, Self-Compassion.org[5], as well as guided self-compassion meditations.

I also like the offerings of Neff's colleague, Dr. Chris Germer. Here is one of his longer videos, specific to shame, "Self-Compassion: An Antidote to Shame"[6], but you can easily find his shorter ones, or those of other therapists.

And if you want to move beyond self-compassion, you can power up to Kristin Neff's book, *FIERCE Self-Compassion: How Women Can Harness Kindness to Speak up, Claim their Power and Thrive.*

Again, self-compassion turbo-boosted my healing and was just as, or perhaps more profound than psychedelics, support groups, somatics and talk therapy. It is one of the most under-rated, yet scientifically proven, tools for healing from trauma and its symptoms.

PART FOUR
SOMATICS

CHAPTER 17
A STRANGE NEW WORLD
(A TITLE BORROWED FROM LEVINE, WAKING THE TIGER)

"Most trauma therapies address the mind through talk, and the molecules of the mind with drugs. Both of these approaches can be of use. However, trauma is not, will not, and can never be fully healed until we also address the essential role played by the body."
– Peter Levine, *Waking the Tiger* (pg. 3)

TBH, I don't fully understand how trauma gets trapped in our bodies and how somatics help to release or resolve it. I can follow the complex explanations of Levine, Maté, van der Kolk and others to a certain degree, but at some point my feeble mind can't keep up and I jump ahead to the more easily understandable conclusions. Like many other areas of my life, I trust the experts.

Somatics is a term used in trauma therapy and is based on the soma, or "the body as perceived from within." Somatic therapy explores how the body expresses overwhelming or painful experiences and how working with the body can be a way of processing and releasing the pain.

A somatic therapist helps people release damaging pent-up emotions held in their body by using a range of mind-body techniques. These can vary widely, ranging from yoga, eye movement, meditation and breathwork to acupressure and dance. More examples later.

Practitioners of somatic therapy view the mind and body as inherently linked. They also believe that trauma can get trapped inside our bodies and affect our physical health, mental health and behavior.

As my wonderful therapist Matthew Gardner said to me in one of our many helpful sessions:

> *"I'm going to try to put it in a nutshell for you. Think about your window of emotional regulation. Within this range you can tolerate and process your emotions. If emotions get too high, you hyper-arouse and get sucked into the trauma vortex. If they get too low, you hypo-arouse, numb out, shut down and dissociate. Either way, you're not present. The reason why so much of our trauma comes from our infancy and childhood is because kids have a narrower window of emotional regulation, because they have fewer coping skills, more fragile nervous systems, and less agency. They don't have the capacity to tolerate their big emotions. Healing happens when we open up those old files, and allow the dysregulated emotions to move through our adult nervous systems that can handle them. Most of the somatic strategies are methods of accessing our own backlog of pain, and staying regulated as we metabolize those emotions so that they don't retraumatize us."*

Peter Levine points out that throughout history, particularly in the east, healthcare had for thousands of years been focused on how the mind affects the body (e.g. psychosomatic medicine), and how every part of the body was represented somewhere in the mind. However, this unity of mind and body has somehow faded in our modern western trauma treatments.

Bessel van der Kolk, meanwhile, distinguishes that body-based therapy is different than talk therapy, and applauds how sensorimotor and somatic therapies acknowledge the body-mind connection:

"In these treatment approaches the story of what has happened takes a backseat to exploring physical sensations and discovering the location and shape of the imprints of past trauma on the body."
– Bessel van der Kolk, *The Body Keeps the Score*
(pg. 219)

So it may seem bizarre that moving our bodies can be key to resolving our trauma and releasing pent up emotions, but the effects have proven to be dramatic.

CHAPTER 18
HYPE OR HOPE? DO SOMATICS WORK?

"The good news is that we don't have to live with it - at least not forever. Trauma can be healed, and even more easily prevented."
– Peter Levine, *Waking the Tiger* (pg 41)

The titles of many books, courses and videos sound too good to be true:

- The Secret to Healing Trauma
- Heal Yourself
- Unbound
- Heal from Within
- Six Ways to Heal Trauma Without Medication
- The Seven Surprising Ways to Heal Trauma Without Medication

I had spent a lot of time wondering if somatics would help me to heal my trauma but remained stuck in a back eddy of skepticism and ignorance. A full decade before I got serious about my trauma my psychologist had written a detailed treatment plan which included trauma therapy. I had been told by multiple doctors and therapists since then that I had trauma and needed to deal with it, but the questions remained:

- Do I really have trauma?
- What is trauma anyways?
- So what?
- What are somatics?
- Do they even work?

I now know they work.

Once again, I am delighted by Dr. Pooky Knightsmith's candid exploration of key concepts that would be helpful for people to know before they start trauma therapy. Although she is speaking specifically about the somatic tool Eye Movement Desensitization and Reprocessing (EMDR), the principles she raises apply to most areas of trauma therapy and somatics:

1. I wish I'd known it was going to work,
2. I wish I'd know it would get worse before it got better, and
3. I wish I'd known I wouldn't have to say it all aloud,

She shares that when EMDR was suggested to her she was in a really bad place, feeling hopeless, and reluctant to try something new because if it didn't work it could potentially take her to an even worse place. If she had known it was going to work it would have instilled greater hope during the initial stages when, as is common, challenges arose.

Decades before others joined the chorus to proclaim the wonders of somatics, Peter Levine was somewhat of a lone prophet; his cries from the wilderness offering promise and hope:

"Having spent the last 25 years working with people who have been

traumatized in almost every conceivable fashion, I believe that we humans have the innate capacity to heal not only ourselves, but our world, from the debilitating effects of trauma."
– Peter Levine, *Waking the Tiger* (pg. 21)

And the preaching continues: "Good news", Maté proclaims in this video. He states that our wounds can be healed and we can be restored.

"Gabor Maté - Trauma Is Not What Happens to You, It Is What Happens Inside You"[1]

Some more motivation from Peter Levine acknowledges that even though everyone has lived through trauma, and there are many symptoms of it, this is not a life sentence. Even in people with more severe instances, such as those suffering from obvious cases of post-traumatic stress, it can be healed, and often prevented. He encourages us to let our "natural, biological instincts" guide us to accomplishing this goal and understanding ourselves in new ways.

Many of us start off with little experience or understanding of the benefits of somatics; however, I encourage you to ignite a small flickering flame of hope, optimism, and perhaps even faith, that they *will* work, as they have for so many others.

CHAPTER 19

VOOO, SPHINCTER CONTRACTIONS, AND EAR MASSAGE

Some of the somatic practices, movements, and methodologies may seem strange and peculiar. Like I once was, you may be hesitant to try them for a number of reasons:

- Most of us are unfamiliar with them. Somatics is a fairly new field of study and research and many are unfamiliar with the practices and postures.
- The benefits are hard to measure. It is difficult to connect a particular movement to a certain improvement or substantial change in health.
- Improvements happen slowly.
- While Western medicine has become increasingly aware of the body-mind connection, it has yet to make its way fully into convention.

Let me put out a bit of a challenge. If a 60-year-old ex-pastor, ex-rugby player, middle-class, father of four, sit-on-the couch boomer can give this stuff a shot, then perhaps you can too.

I'll start with a few of the stranger sounding exercises just to get your attention, then list a few others:

THE VOO SOUND

I was quite eager to watch this YouTube video as the renowned Peter Levine is providing instruction: "A Simple Exercise to Ease Despair with Peter Levine, PhD" | *NICABM*[1]. In it, Levine gives instructions on how to alleviate strong feelings of despair by using a simple but powerful exercise. I was really surprised at the simplicity and strangeness of this exercise and to hear a world-renowned trauma specialist demonstrate it for us. To do this exercise you take a deep inhale, then make a vooo sound that emanates from the base of your belly until all the breath is exhaled.

Although I use this exercise often and find it to be beneficial, at first, I was surprised and doubtful because I thought it was, well, weird.

SPHINCTER CONTRACTIONS

In this YouTube video, "How to Stimulate Your Vagus Nerve and Why You Should Try It"[2], Deepak Chopra, states that contracting and expanding the sphincter muscle will stimulate the vagus nerve. You can do this while sitting or lying on your back, either with your bum on the floor, or with knees raised and your bum a few inches off the floor. I know, it seems crazy! But apparently it works. I sometimes do it in combination with the vooo sound, and/or EMDR. Yup, things are getting strange – but I think it's helping me.

EAR MASSAGE

The last of the stranger-sounding exercises I want to direct your attention to is ear massage. The following YouTube video by Sukie Baxter, "Vagus Nerve Massage For Stress And Anxiety Relief"[3] introduces it quite well. The point of the ear massage is to stimulate the Vagus nerve which has been shown to send messages to the brain that relieve depression and anxiety, and alter mood.

Personally, my definition for somatics is quite broad. If a practice is affecting or involves any of my bodily senses, and I am being mindful or intentional to involve my mind, then I think of it as somatic. But it may be helpful to see these tools, activities and methodologies as falling into three general groupings; somatics, semi-somatics, and non-somatics.

These are activities that I personally practice or have practiced. These are not exhaustive lists. Van der Koch, Maté, and Levine list a variety of other modalities and techniques that I am not going to review. Obviously, they can be found in their books and videos.

At times, I have been guided by therapists and coaches, but currently do my practices by myself and sometimes with friends (other than yoga with a group, and massage with a RMT or masseuse).

SOMATICS

- Sauna
- Cold immersion
- Breathwork
- Yoga
- Hot yoga
- Ocean/sunlight/wave therapy
- Massage
- Lacrosse ball self-massage
- Vooo sound
- EMDR
- Vibration therapy
- Sound bath
- Vagus nerve stimulation

- Sphincter contraction
- Aroma therapy

SEMI-SOMATIC

- Meditation
- Drumming
- Tibetan Singing bowl
- Body Intuitive
- Singing
- Writing
- Laughing
- Dancing
- Psychedelics/Plant medicine
- Acupuncture
- Forest bathing

NON-SOMATIC

- Listening to music
- Self-compassion
- Forgiveness/Resentments and Fears
- Prayer and meditation
- Affirmations
- Reading or listening to audio books

Some somatic practices on these lists (here or earlier) may seem odd or completely bizarre, but give them a shot to determine what works for you.

CHAPTER 20
THE SHAKING BEAR

S haking or trembling is an interesting side effect that individuals experiencing energetic trauma release sometimes encounter.

Emotions get trapped in the body because, after a traumatic event, the nervous system quickly resorts to survival mode - fight, flight or freeze. The idea is that in this state, stress hormones are continually released. When the body is under this constant level of stress, physical and psychological symptoms emerge.

Somatic therapy practitioners point to the phenomenon of animals shaking off their trauma and stress after scares, like nearly being eaten, in order to 'move through' the danger. This response calms their nervous system and quiets the 'fight or flight' response.

While watching the 1982 National Geographic video "Polar Bear Alert" Peter Levine observed the trembling and spontaneous shaking of a polar bear waking up after being shot with a tranquilizer dart. This observation became a catalytic moment in his development of somatic theory.

Around the 11:00 minute mark of this video, "Nature's Lessons in Healing Trauma: An Introduction to Somatic Experiencing"[1],

Levine shows the famous shaking polar bear video that was a catalyst in the formation of his early theories around somatics.

It is remarkable that Levine's revelations occurred during the normal flow of life as he watched nature shows on television. Also remarkable is how by looking at our connection to other mammals, Levine was able to make significant breakthroughs. I find this use of basic reasoning and a common sense approach to be encouraging, refreshing and easy to understand.

Interestingly, trembling and shaking also sometimes occurs during psychedelic assisted trauma therapy. As an article in the Psychedelic.Support website titled "Can Psychedelics Help Us Release Trauma Through Shaking?"[2] states:

"It is common for many people to find themselves shaking, trembling, shivering, or spasming during a psychedelic experience. This is often reported as involuntary, coming out of nowhere. But it can feel like a kind of release, leading to a state of euphoria and calm."

I believe that breakthroughs in physical and emotional healing can also occur as we read or listen to transformative information. I have felt physical reactions in my body as I heard a paradigm-shifting statement while listening to an audio book. On one of those occasions while driving, I had a powerful recurring leg twitch simultaneous to the mind-jarring mental stimulation.

Cognitive illumination can result in physical transformation. Perhaps these serendipitous realizations, or "aha moments", can result in bursts of energetic healing in my body.

It encourages me to be aware and attentive to indicators and information from a variety of sources. I am not saying every TV show, conversation or random piece of data has some special meaning or significance. Neither am I saying that when I do pick up a helpful nudge or guidance from a novel source that I should use "Hans-logic" to inflate it into some kind of divinely inspired theory with grandiose purpose.

Some therapists suggest that intentionally shaking our bodies can replicate the natural trembling response and release trauma. In this YouTube video Emma McAdam, a licensed marriage and family therapist provides some background to her theory and suggests some intentional body shaking: "How to Release Emotions Trapped in Your Body 10/30 How to Process Emotions Like Trauma and Anxiety"[3].

Try to see if you can find your own accounts in the online community: YouTube, Facebook, Reddit, etc. Here's one I found on Reddit that spoke to me:

 Been shaking and tremoring for a while, but still no emotions?

Remain curious and open to learning about somatics from a variety of sources. And don't be alarmed if you experience sudden sensations, such as shaking or trembling as you undergo phases of healing and transformation.

CHAPTER 21
EMDR

This joke I like to say about EMDR comes across a lot better when said in person than in writing, but this attempt at humor actually has a point.

The acronym EMDR stands for the tongue-twisting 14 syllable phrase:

(Eye) I Was In The Park and Felt Better When I Moved My Eyes

Just kidding, EMDR actually stands for *Eye Movement Desensitization and Reprocessing.*

The point of my silly word play is to highlight the fact that what has become a proven therapy had humble beginnings. As humble as a walk in the park.

For a number of reasons, which I will get to later, it is worth noting EMDR's genesis:

In 1987, Francine Shapiro was walking in the park when she realized that eye movements appeared to decrease the negative emotion associated with her own distressing memories.

In the YouTube video, "EMDR interview Francine Shapiro"[1],

she describes the genesis and development of this therapy. It is note-worthy that after the host asks her guest how she discovered EMDR, Shapiro tosses her head back and chuckles before answering, as if to indicate the novelty and unconventionality of her initial experience.

"Well it actually began 10 years before the discovery when I got cancer, and it changed the work I was doing on a PhD in English literature and put the concentration on mind and body.
...so I began to use my mind and body as a laboratory to explore these interventions and techniques. One day I was walking along and I noticed that some disturbing thoughts I was having were suddenly disappearing. I noticed that when those thoughts came through my mind that my eyes started moving very rapidly in a certain way."

Well the rest is history. EMDR is now a structured therapy that encourages the patient to focus briefly on the trauma memory while simultaneously being directed to move their eyes back and forth. EMDR therapy is an extensively researched, effective psychotherapy method proven to help people recover from trauma and PTSD symptoms. Ongoing research supports positive clinical outcomes showing EMDR therapy as a helpful treatment for disorders such as anxiety, depression, OCD, chronic pain, addictions, and other distressing life experiences. EMDR therapy has even been superior to Prozac in trauma treatment. More than 7 million people have been treated successfully by 110,000 therapists in 130 countries since 2016.

The elements of Shapiro's wonderful discovery that stand out for me are:

- Her own cancer diagnosis prompted her to seek a remedy.
- She was using her own mind and body as a laboratory and exploring techniques.
- She was walking in the park, not sitting in a lab.

- She noticed an improvement in her own troubling thoughts.
- She took action further to this somewhat bizarre revelation.
- She patiently applied analysis and scientific principles to validate her theory.
- It has become a proven therapy that has brought relief to millions around the world.

Take a walk in the park. Who knows what you may learn?

CHAPTER 22
INTERGENERATIONAL SOMATICS

"If you cannot get rid of the family skeleton, you may as well make it dance."
– George Bernard Shaw

For the most part, I have endeavored to only include material in this book that is evidence-based or sourced from the writings and practices of credible trauma specialists and practitioners. The following offering is more theoretical and based on the theories that have crossed my mind as I have read and practiced somatics and worked to resolve my trauma.

As I describe earlier, I am fascinated by Peter Levine's accounts of significant moments of illumination and discovery occurring while he simply watched animal behavior on television nature shows. From there, with curiosity and passion he used reason and common sense to develop suppositions and theories. I am sure some of his colleagues thought these ideas to be far-reaching or even far-fetched, but they became the foundation for therapy that is practiced and taught world-wide today.

Similarly, Francine Shapiro organically stumbled upon EMDR

while walking in a park and dealing with personal distressing thoughts. But the fertile ground for that scene was established years earlier when she had switched her studies to focus on mind-body medicine due to a cancer diagnosis. She then informally tested theories and methodologies by using her mind and body as a living laboratory. Fascinating!

Levine and Shapiro's willingness to think outside the box and imagine unique solutions is inspiring. They were curious, courageous, and creative. As I suggest in Part 3 - You Are Your Own Guide, it may be necessary for those of us seeking wellness to muster some imagination, curiosity and creativity. Additionally, like Shapiro, we can test methodologies and use our mind and bodies as living laboratories in an effort to determine what works best for ourselves, and perhaps others.

In this spirit of creativity and experiment I have been practicing something I call intergenerational somatics. I also refer to it synonymously as generational somatics or ancestral somatics. My reasoning behind it is based on the extensive writing of Gabor Maté and others regarding intergenerational trauma, which I touch on elsewhere.

In the last couple of years I have entered into what Peter Levine calls a 'strange new land,' and developed a somatic practice in an effort to resolve trauma—perhaps including intergenerational trauma. Over this period some questions came to mind:

- If harm or negative consequences can cross generations, then isn't it reasonable that helpful and positive influences are available intergenerationally?
- If trauma can be passed from one generation to the next, then is it possible that there are opportunities to reverse or resolve that trauma that are also intergenerational in nature?
- Could there be somatic practices, movements, and physical, mental and emotional activities that my ancestors practiced that would be therapeutic for me?

- Are there movements or mind-body activities that were unique to my predecessors, as opposed to someone else's predecessors?
- Were there somatic experiences in my lineage that were linked to moments of peace, security, safety and meaningful connection? In other words, healing?

These ponderings have led me to some regular experimental practices which I feel are helping me. I am still a work in progress, but some of my symptoms have subsided completely, and others are becoming less severe.

THE OLD MAN AND THE SEA

Currently, I live in a beautiful waterfront location. The cold waters of the Strait of Juan de Fuca are right across the street, 25 meters from my front door. My living room window is south facing and looks over the Strait with the mountains of the Olympic Peninsula standing majestic before me. I can sit and look out that window for hours. I have had many ups and downs over the last year - good days and bad - but no matter what, the view feels calming and healing.

As I write this, I am thinking that I should probably try to paint an elaborate word-picture with descriptors and superlatives that make the reader feel like they are personally experiencing my view of the waves, sunlight, ships, birds etc. But I'm not going to do that. Fancy prose and descriptors won't work. I want to convey something simple, deep in my gut, primal:

I just feel really good when I look at the ocean.

And I'm pretty sure my ancestors did too. My father was born in the small coastal town Langesund, Norway, and was descended from a long line of sea-farers. His father and mother, Farfar and Farmor to me (father's-father and father's-mother), spent their later years in a

Skipperhus (Skipper House), a retirement home for those who worked aboard Norway's famous fleet of ships and freighters.

As far back as my relatives recall, the males on my father's side went to sea. Farfar, Isak Anderssen, sailed on the whaling ships that harvested in the southern Arctic Ocean, as did his father. Nordic seafaring in my family can be traced right back to the explorations and conquests of the fearless Vikings. Okay, maybe my Viking-ness exists only in my wildly grandiose imagination.

An interesting side-note on my whaling heritage. I have hiked the West Coast trail, a six-day, 75 km rough coastal trail on Vancouver Island three times, and each time I always seem to be the first one in our hiking group to spot the blow-hole spray from the migrating gray whales off shore. My wife asked me why I was always looking for whales. I came to realize that it wasn't intentional, I was just naturally drawn to look out over the ocean. Without thinking, I was intuitively glancing out to sea. Just like my ancestors, I suppose.

So does it stand to reason that in my physiology or mind-body, there is some kind of connection to the sea? As my ancestors looked out to sea, gazed at the ocean, checked the wind and waves or traveled and toiled at sea, what was happening in their minds? Would they not have experienced feelings of sustenance, fulfillment, prosperity, exhilaration, adventure and security? The sea brought their food, their loved ones, trade goods, and social connection. Their physical activities centered around the sea; fishing, moving cargo, maintaining boats, nets and gear. Their minds, bodies and overall well being were linked indivisibly to the ocean. Did my Norwegian ancestors unknowingly practice what I call ocean-based psychosomatics?

I am sure most people find the ocean therapeutic to some degree, but could it be a form of deeper Somatic Experiencing for those of us with a lineage anchored to the sea?

I think of my sons, whose ocean-based legacy is perhaps even stronger than mine. Their great grandfather on their mother's side, Alexander Ranalla, was the most successful and notorious bootlegger on the Baltic Sea in the 1930's and 40's. He lived in Estonia and had such a powerful boat that he could outrun the authorities as he made his daring runs across the Baltic to Finland with booze where the Finns - who are known to enjoy a drink or two - suffered under prohibition.

Adding to this swashbuckling tale is the outlandishly romantic account of him being enamoured with a pretty Finn-Swede girl (there is an area in southern Finland populated by Swedes) named Ines who was admiring this legendary treasure-laden sea-farer from the dock as he unloaded his cargo. On a later trip he proposed, married her, and brought her back to Viinistu, Estonia, a small coastal village where they had three sons, including Ivor Ranalla, my sons' grandfather.

The connection to the ocean is deeply embedded in my sons' heritage. Could it benefit them somatically as well?

Perhaps my "generational ocean-based somatics" theory is only romantic speculation. Perhaps it is foolish of me to think it is particularly beneficial for me and others with seafaring in their genealogy. But interestingly, studies show that ocean-based therapy can be healing. An article published on Medical Bag.com titled "Ocean Therapy Has the Power to Heal the Mind and Body"[1] explains how soldiers suffering from PTSD benefited from surfing.

OCEAN-BASED SOMATICS

I have always loved the ocean, but never really thought about it from an ancestral perspective. I had a fish boat for a few years and was obsessed with fishing. The improvement in my mental health and emotional well-being in those years was noticeable.

I'm not out fishing very often lately so these days my ocean therapy includes the following (I am not suggesting my ancestors did these exact activities [they didn't have access to the YouTube videos because the internet connection was shitty]). I have morphed contemporary somatic exercises together with my ancestral connection to the sea:

- Ocean viewing with meditation and mindfulness
- Cold immersion
- Coastal hikes and exercise (Regular 30 minute "Viking run" - beach, logs, rocks)
- Oceanside breathwork or breathwork during cold immersion
- Oceanside EMDR, or EMDR during cold immersion
- Ocean side sunlight therapy; can also be done during cold immersion
- Earthing/grounding on sand or rocks
- Oceanside or cold immersion combined with one of the following: Voo sound, self-compassion, or Vagus nerve massage
- Paddle boarding with mindfulness/meditation

Recently, I had a surprising somatic experience while walking in the soft pre-dawn light on a wooden wharf on Northern Vancouver Island where a fleet of commercial fishing boats were moored. As I crossed the planks in my rubber boots, imperceptible vibrations seemed to pass through my entire body, bringing me comfort and serenity. Misty rain fell, seagulls circled and the smell of the sea and fish boats touched all my senses.

Realizing my Felt Sense, as Peter Levine calls it, was perceiving something, I imagined that I was walking in the footsteps of my ancestors. Then - and this might seem a little woo-woo - but it's a true story, I came around the bow of a boat and smiled when I saw its name; "Alta Viking". Alta is a coastal town in Norway. And I think I mentioned my boyishly fantastical Viking connections. Coincidence or woo-woo?

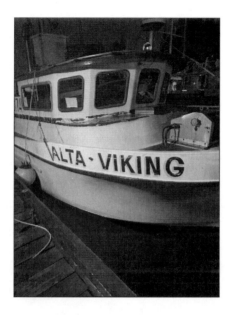

In addition to ocean-based somatics, I am practicing other somatic, semi-somatic, and non-somatic activities and also exploring a wide variety of healing modalities. I have noticed significant improvements in my health but I believe that it is due to doing many things in combination - not just the ocean therapy, or any other single modality. For me, there is no one silver bullet or magic potion.

MOUNTAIN SOMATICS AND CARPENTRY SOMATICS

I also enjoy a rich connection to the mountains and forests on my mother's side. My Morfar, built a lodge in the mountains north of Oslo that they called Viderheim, which I believe translates as 'far-away home'.

There is a legendary tale that is well known amongst my mother's family. My grandfather was alone at Viderheim, chopping wood for the stove. The sharp axe somehow glanced off the wood and sunk deep into his lower leg. He was bleeding profusely and the nearest village was many kilometers away. He needed to get to help, but would not survive the long hike with blood pouring from the wound.

Fortunately, Mormor had left some sewing supplies at the cabin and he found a large needle and a spool of wool. What makes this tale more legendary is that the wool was red. Imagine my Morfar sewing up his own leg with no freezing or anesthetic, hiking over the mountains, and arriving in the village with his leg sewn up with red yarn.

Despite the wood-chopping accident, my father was a skilled carpenter and I was able to visit Viderheim and see his carpentry shop and old tools in the out-building.

So maybe I am stretching things, but is it a coincidence that I love being in the mountains and also enjoy doing carpentry. Over the years we have taken our four boys on countless day-hikes, and each summer made sure to do at least one multi-day back-packing adventure on the rugged coast or high in the mountains.

Although physically exhausted after a 5 day hike, it is difficult to put into words the inner contentment and peace that I enjoy - deep somatic healing. Additionally our familial and social connection was strengthened. This past summer, my boys and I climbed the highest viewable peak in the Olympic range that I see out my front window across the Juan de Fuca strait.

I am not a skilled carpenter but get a kick out of building a sauna or a whimsical coffee table. And remember Morfar chopping wood at Viderheim? That is an activity that for me feels both meditative and primal - and I'm pretty sure, somatic. Chopping wood is at the same time both exhausting and intrinsically replenishing. I am replicating a physical action going back far more than seven generations.

I wonder what the subconscious thoughts in my ancestors mind and emotions would be? A visceral sense of security - *chop* - safety - *chop* - fuel for cooking - *chop* - sustenance - *chop* - comfort - *chop* - "my family is safe". I picture my Morfar's Morfar stopping to wipe the sweat from his brow as he views the growing wood pile with primal contentment and deep fulfillment. Somatic therapy.

Psychoneuroimmunology was the same for them as it is for me. The human body has not changed. We just have fancy scientific terms now. I would love to know the somatic mind-body benefits of chopping wood.

WHERE DID YOUR ANCESTORS LIVE?

A parallel thought to ancestral somatics is the idea of land-based somatics. Friends who grew up on the prairies have told me how peaceful and relaxed they feel when they return home. Gazing out over a field as the wind blows the grain and the clouds move across an endless sky is like therapy for them.

I met an Irishman once who went on and on (God bless the Irish, but they can talk!) describing the beauty of being born and raised in a small village on a beautiful river. I wonder if his somatic genealogy would be different from me or my prairie friend.

What about the person from a tropical country, or the arctic, or a village high in the Andes? Are there land-based activities or experiences that could enhance their mind-body wellness? I am only speculating, but perhaps these thoughts will aid someone in their quest for healing.

I stumbled across a very short snippet in a conversation between Alianis Morissette and Peter Levine that touches on land-based somatics. "Episode 8 - Conversation with Alanis Morissette & Dr. Peter Levine"[2]. It is a quick tangential exchange and I almost missed it. It could be that I am reading way too much into it but I believe it is note-worthy:

> Levine: "I was doing my graduate work on medical biophysics at Berkeley and I happened to go down to Big Sur for a weekend."
> Morissette: "And a swim?"
> Levine: "And a swim. And I realized this was more interesting, so I took a leave of absence."

Morissette: "Interesting because of how sensual and somatic that is."
Levine: "Ahhh, primal! Primal land. It's a powerful land."
Morissette: "Rugged."

Interesting that Morissette pointed out the somatics of the land and Levine emphatically agreed, "Ahh, primal! Primal land. It's a powerful land."

"If trauma can be inherited from one generation to the next, then so can love, emotional intelligence and wisdom."
- Anonymous

WHAT DID GRANDMA DO?

It's not rocket surgery! Our ancestors have been doing somatics of various sorts for centuries:

- for survival
- for sustenance
- for enjoyment
- for recreation
- for social interaction
- as part of daily, weekly and seasonal routine

Ask your ancestors, God, Creator, and yourself:

- What did your grandparents, great grandparents and ancestors do that brought them health?
- What did they do physically, somatically, mentally and emotionally?
- What activities and influences have gone into your design?

The experts tell us that the effects of trauma can be passed on from generation to generation. Surely there has to be a positive side to our ancestral connections that lightens the burdens that we have inherited.

"The universe wants to heal us. The universe is emanating love. We need to find out what is blocking the love. What hinders us."
— Sumi

PART FIVE
PSYCHEDELICS

CHAPTER 23
ALL THE KING'S HORSES

"As a modality of healing, it is beyond insane that these things are illegal."
– Gabor Maté

There is an old Gary Larson, Far Side comic I really like. Unfortunately, for copyright reasons my editor won't let me put it in this book, so here is an attempt to explain it. First off, you have to be old enough to remember the nursery rhyme,

"Humpty Dumpty sat on a wall. Humpty Dumpty had a great fall. All the King's horses and all the King's men, couldn't put Humpty together again."

So, here is the tedious description of the Far Side comic: The soldiers are standing around a cracked and broken egg-shaped Humpty. Behind them some horses are standing on their hind legs looking impatiently as the soldiers try unsuccessfully to fix Humpty. One of the soldiers says "Ok, Ok, you guys have had your chance. The horses want another shot at it."

Ba-da-bum.

When the students in Bessel van der Kolk's psychedelic drug research lab excitedly claim to be part of *the* psychedelic revolution, he correctively reminds them that they are part of *the second* revolution. The first revolution occurred when these drugs were being studied with positive results by Timothy Leary and other respected scientists (btw, Bill Wilson, who had founded Alcoholics Anonymous decades earlier, participated in experiments with Leary to address his depression).

Unfortunately, this promising research of 60 years ago ended, at least in part, due to the misclassification and grouping of these substances with addictive narcotics, the international effects of Nixon's 'War on Drugs', and the pharmaceutical industry's lack of interest in funding clinical trials.

Fortunately, a second revolution is upon us, and in a few years psychedelics will be a part of mainstream mental health care. But progress is painfully slow, and as we wait, I whole-heartedly agree with Gabor Maté who states, "As a modality of healing, it is beyond insane that these things are illegal."

So, to awkwardly close out my Hans-splaining the Far Side comic: psychedelics are like the King's horses impatiently waiting for another chance to fix things. It's really un-funny to write out an explanation for a comic. Blech. Oh, well. I just could not let go of it - I had to get that comic into this book somehow. I'm pretty sure it is vital to everything else making any sense.

Psychedelics have a troubled past but significant effort is being made to change the paradigm and perspective around these helpful medicines. Psychedelic drugs have long been an accepted part of many of the world's cultures and altered states of consciousness have been integrated into communities in most civilizations other than the West for thousands of years.

Psychedelics are hallucinogenic drugs[1] that can change our mental state and affect our consciousness. Psychedelics can cause one to think, see and hear things that are out of our normal realm of experience.

I suppose it is to be expected that when I mention psychedelics people respond with either a wry half-smile and mention something about high-school or college, or say something polite and proper like "oh, interesting" as they glance around to make sure their children are kept away from the druggie in the room.

If you are unfamiliar with the use of psychedelics for the treatment of trauma and mental health issues, I encourage you to consider whether you carry unhelpful bias, stereotypes or stigma towards them. Disdain, erroneous perceptions and close-mindedness may hinder your openness to considering them as a helpful medical tool.

I write more about cross-cultural communication and removing unhelpful stereotypes elsewhere.

But change is underway as researchers and medical professionals, driven by the evidence supporting the benefits of psychedelics, focus on altering the narrative. Psychedelics will be part of mainstream medical treatment in the next few years. The evidence for their efficacy, after countless studies at the top research institutions throughout the world, is indisputable.

My curiosity about psychedelics was piqued years ago when I first heard Gabor Maté mention his experiences with ayahuasca. The whole psychedelic culture seemed weird and unattractive to me, but I was intrigued that a respected medical expert was openly promoting psychedelic plant medicine and Shamanistic ceremonies birthed in the Amazonian jungle. At the time I had no inclination or desire to participate personally.

Then in 2021, after a particularly challenging period, I began to aggressively investigate unconventional treatment modalities. I began to hear more and more about the use of psychedelics as a treatment for mental health. Around this time, I finally accepted that I needed to do intensive trauma work, and consider options other than just the conventional talk therapy and the support groups that I had relied on for years which had resulted in some progress but provided only intermittent periods of stability.

As tends to happen to many of us, the message I needed to hear, and the lesson I needed to learn, began to manifest serendipitously through multiple mediums: books, friends, media, therapists, out-of-the-blue conversations, and other unexpected sources. One confirming and encouraging prompt came through conversations with my intelligent, caring, and well-read adult sons.

Around the same time, my wife and one of my sons were both attending the University of Victoria. One 2021 article from UVic News titled, "Psychedelics Revisited"[2], which grabbed my attention, posed the question of whether psychedelics were ready to be part of mainstream mental healthcare in Canada. Doctor Evan Wood commented on the likelihood, stating:

Ready for the mainstream?
In the next four to five years, it's likely that psychedelic-assisted therapy will be part of mainstream mental-health care in Canada, says Wood. It's going to take "private-sector motivation and ingenuity" coupled with leadership from federal policymakers to achieve this.

In the YouTube video "Gabor Maté on Psychedelics, Trauma and the Body (Part 5)"[3], Maté offers that although he believes psychedelics have potential, no one thing has the ability to change the world. He has, however, seen many benefits across health sectors, from trauma to addiction, and even to autoimmune diseases, and advocates for them to be studied and explored more seriously.

I had read and heard Maté's opinion on and promotion of psychedelics in multiple places over the years, but was pleasantly surprised recently when I discovered Bessel van der Kolk also strongly endorses psychedelics.

In the YouTube video "The 7 Surprising Ways To Heal Trauma Without Medication"[4], Dr. Rangan Chaterjee asks van der Kolk to share his views on psychedelics. Van der Kolk's remarks on this subject begin around the 1 hour 15 min point of the video and continue for about 10 minutes. He passionately and enthusiastically promotes psychedelics, but interestingly, with equal passion provides some cautionary advice. Here are a few selected comments:

"This is not just a matter of opinion because my lab now does psychedelic studies and I am really very happy to be part of this burgeoning thing. I have a license to give MDMA/ecstasy, I'm part of a larger study that's almost done, with good data. The only psychedelic that's currently legal in America right now is ketamine, and I'm involved in training people in ketamine assisted psychotherapy".

As I researched 5-MEO DMT and Ibogaine, I connected with and had a very informative phone conversation with Anders Beatty in England who has over 25 years experience in the field of addiction, firstly as an "addict" and later as an addictions coach specializing in plant medicine integration.

Anders founded Ibogaine Counseling Services in England after his own transformative treatment with Ibogaine for cocaine addiction. Anders' pre-treatment protocol has become recognised as a fundamental component of successful treatment by many of the world's leading Ibogaine providers.

In the informative video, "The Real Cause of Drug Addiction...And a Plant Medicine Solution"[5], Anders explains:

"Our success rate with plant medicine in comparison to NA, AA, detox or rehab is, well, we just blow them out of the water completely. Completely blow them out of the water."

And Anders said to me on the phone:

"Hans, I'm not trying to sell you anything or criticize any other recovery or healing modalities, but I was a committed member of NA and AA, attended meetings for years, had probably 8 or 9 sponsors -

and finally reached a point where I realized that trying to do a more thorough step 4, or worrying I had missed an amends on my step 9 was not going to keep me clean and sober. Plant medicine provided a breakthrough for me."

Eventually, in my Viking-esque desire for exploration, I decided to pursue psychedelic-assisted therapy. So far my treatment has included LSD, psilocybin, ayahuasca, and 5-MeO-DMT. I also applied for and was accepted into a ketamine research trial, but unfortunately I was unable to participate.

You may be wondering, "How was it? Describe your experiences? What happened?" Well, they have helped me. A lot.

Although I share openly and exuberantly the details of my psychedelic experiences with friends and family, and especially fellow-sufferers seeking healing, I'm hesitant to go into much detail here for a few reasons:

- Experiences can vary widely. While I did extensive research into the safety, protocols, suggested delivery, and general effects of each medicine, I purposefully avoided listening to or reading detailed and vivid accounts. I did not want to taint my own experience with that of someone else, and possibly set myself up for disappointment or confusion. I didn't want "my movie experience" spoiled by someone pre-telling me the scenes in their movie - I established my own "spoiler alert system". If I was going to put significant time, effort, money and energy into these journeys, I wanted my vistas to be pristine and unique.
- The integration or application in the days, weeks and months afterward is more important than the actual medicine event. The time under the medicine is not the purpose or a "moment unto itself". Our objective is long-term change and healing. Focusing on the sensational

and experiential can take away from the greater
questions; "What did that mean? What am I to learn?
How will this bring healing?"

- There are many alternative medicines and psychedelics
  and I don't want my experience with a particular
  medicine to infer that one is better than the other. I
  believe results, benefits and healing may vary person to
  person.
- I take others' healing journeys very seriously and don't
  want a sensational telling of my story regarding a
  particular medicine to either entice or deter anybody.
- Some of my experiences are personal, private, and
  perhaps touching on the sacred.

To be clear, psychedelics were an essential part of my quest for
healing over the last few years and I expect that they will continue to
be. Becoming curious, then open, and eventually embracing them
was a process. I had to shift my world-view, endure the skepticism
and ignorance of others, and do a lot of research. But I took my time
and did not jump into anything impulsively.

You, too, may have biases and misconceptions that are hindering
you from considering psychedelics. As you overcome these historical
stigmas, take the time you need to consider the benefits and implications these medicines may have for you.

CHAPTER 24
MY EXPERIENCE WITH PSILOCYBIN

I think it might be helpful for me to share some details from one medicinal application, and the mistakes I made following that experience.

My therapists have identified transgenerational, prenatal, childhood, and adult experiences of trauma that occurred on various levels: physical, emotional, psychological, and religious. I recall feeling a mix of surprise, disappointment and relief when my psychologist told me I scored 7 out of 10 on the Adverse Childhood Experiences (ACEs) Questionnaire.

I don't go into detail about the details of my trauma in this book because I never meant for it to be a memoir or primarily autobiographical. I have included the following account with the goal of illustrating how psychedelics can open the door to understanding and resolving past events.

While other elements, situations and occurrences in my life were more damaging to me, a traumatic event that impacted me was the death of one of my sisters at the age of 17, when I was 11 years old. I was at a summer camp an hour away from home when my 4 sisters were in a car accident late on a summer night.

Although there were still 3 days remaining in my week at camp, late that night the camp director woke me up and in a somber hushed tone told me that my parents wanted me to return home after breakfast the next morning. After breakfast I was silently trundled into the car of a volunteer cabin leader, a close friend of my older brother. He didn't talk much as we drove back to Victoria and he had the radio on to break the awkward silence. No information whatsoever of what had happened to my sisters had been shared with me.

As we drove the news came on the radio stating that there had been a car accident the previous night involving four sisters from Victoria - one of them, Lene Anderssen, had died.

Both the driver and I remained silent, staring ahead at the road. I suppose I immediately entered some kind of shock or denial response since, although I clearly heard that my sister had died, I didn't react. I was driven to the hospital, and there my parents, obviously grief-stricken themselves, gently shared the tragic news.

Because our family was immersed in the theology and world view of conservative religion, in the following days and weeks, natural emotion and grief was suppressed. I listened to church leaders and adults God-'splaining the accident, and offering obtuse phrases which were intended to comfort but instead implanted confusion and anger.

Fast forward forty plus years, and I am lying on a bed after drinking a tasty concoction of berry tea, honey, ginger and a macrodose of psilocybin. In the weeks prior I had multiple meetings with my pioneering and compassionate therapist, Anne-Marie Armour, in preparation for the medicine session. I have an eye-covering mask and earphones on to remove external stimulation. Under the care and guidance of both her and an assistant, I enter an unbelievable 3-4 hour journey into the hidden but very real and relevant recesses of my mind and memories.

Early in this session I perceive the drawers of a dusty file cabinet pulled open. Fingers knowingly flipped through thousands of old files and precisely pulled out certain ones - each with vivid pictures and relevant information from my past:

I am 11 years old, in the car coming home from camp when the news came on the radio. This time, as I heard my sister's name, I did not slip into immediate shock, denial or suppression of my emotions. I burst into tears and wailed - the grief and raw emotion of an 11-year-old boy pouring out of my system - unlocked after 49 years - the dam broken, the pain released. I don't know how long that period of full body, mind and emotional release went on. It felt so good - I recall feeling in-the-moment relief together with the release of ancient unresolved pain.

Then I began to have an amazing revelation and a beautiful new perspective of the unimaginable trauma, grief and sadness that my parents and siblings experienced.

My sisters, physically and emotionally traumatized, pulled out of the wreck, the screams, bodies and blood embedded in their memories.

The hospitals, surgeries, wheelchairs; months and years of physical recovery and survivor's guilt.

Also, my two older brothers: I entered into the sense of their pain, scars, and crippling memories. Nineteen and twenty-two years old - stoic, strong young men - carrying our family's burdens - looking out for and protecting their sisters - and protecting me.

And remarkably, my parents came into view. I saw them as fellow adults. Younger then than I was now. Losing a daughter, their beloved family fractured, broken - the agony must have been so, so deep. I observed their feelings of responsibility and even shame. All compounded by the reality of a loving church community, but a theology composed of mixed messages that can lead to unexpressed pain and repressed emotion.

I felt so much compassion, understanding and sympathy flooding over me. My poor parents, brothers and sisters. As I entered into their personal stories and trauma around this tragedy, I felt freedom and relief - in addition to deep compassion and empathy.

There were many other beautiful substories that came to me

during my time with this medicine, but in the weeks following I made some serious errors. I did not take the necessary time to process or learn how to sort through the messages, gifts and teachings of my time with the medicine.

This essential phase in post-medicine healing is called integration. I was so enthused and excited by my first psychedelic experience that within 2 weeks, against my therapist's advice, I entered a week-long training course to enable me to guide and assist others.

I wrongly assumed the bulk of my personal work had been completed during my medicinal experience. It had impacted me so greatly that I assumed the healing I was seeking had taken place. I was wrong. I came to realize that just like heart surgery or knee replacement, months of rehabilitation were required. Learning to walk again after such radical surgery, reopening and realignment is a slow process.

While I did not lose the raw recollection and benefit of the experience, I had to learn how to apply and adapt to what I had received before my symptoms subsided. As I mentioned elsewhere, it often gets worse before it gets better. It did for me. Much worse.

A NEW APPROACH TO PSILOCYBIN-ASSISTED THERAPY

People may have various reasons for wanting to macro-dose psilocybin (macro-dosing is typically 4 - 6.5 grams, takes 6 to 8 hours, and includes 2 attendants). When I help people who are interested in psilocybin I suggest three possible approaches to this medicine.

1. Recreational or curiosity

- The individual is not experiencing a crisis or processing trauma. They want to try psilocybin in a safe setting.
- One preparatory phone call before treatment, and one follow-up call after is usually sufficient.

- A therapist and assistant guide and assist you during the session.

2. Personal growth, wellness, or "small 't' trauma"

- The individual wants change - but isn't in crisis. E.g. career, relationships, feeling stuck, lack of fulfillment, creativity breakthrough, spiritual exploration, relationship to food, alcohol or substances (not full-on addiction), behaviours, recovery booster.
- Usually one preparatory/intention setting session is appropriate and one or two integration sessions are recommended.
- A therapist and assistant guide and assist you during the session.

3. Significant trauma or health issue

- This level of treatment is meant for someone in crisis eg. PTSD, addiction, significant mental health challenges, grief/loss, "big 'T' Trauma", or the existential crisis associated with terminal illness.
- This treatment program is carried out with the involvement or in coordination with a doctor or professional therapist. It includes multiple preparatory sessions and an extensive integration period of multiple months.
- A therapist and assistant guide and assist you during the session.

If I hadn't taken the risk of macro-dosing psilocybin I would have missed out on insights that were key to resolving trauma from my childhood. However, there isn't a one-size-fits-all approach; we need to provide creative models that serve the goals and needs of a variety of people.

I am also aware of many group-based approaches to psychedelic-assisted experiences. There are extensive resources and opportunities to engage with these facilitators. The benefits of a communal approach can be profound.

CHAPTER 25
MY EXPERIENCE WITH
5-MEO-DMT

W hat follows is a general outline of my personal interaction with this medicine. I will not provide details on chemistry, development, or pharmacology. If I tried to do that I would be way out of my lane – I am not a medical professional, nor an expert. Readers should do their own extensive research and follow the guidance of well-informed medical practitioners or therapists, as I did.

I will also not go into detail about the ceremonial, cultural or therapeutic setting and delivery, how I ingested the medicine, the specifics of my experience under the medicine or details of how it impacted me in the long term. These elements vary greatly for different individuals and I do not want my experience to infer specific guidance, nor be a deterrent, to readers.

Also, some of it is quite personal, perhaps even sacred, and difficult to convey. I am happy – and usually quite passionate and excited – to colorfully share the details in smaller and more personal settings, where I feel it is appropriate and beneficial.

My goal is to convey that this medicine was one of the many healing modalities made available to me, and I believe it was an *important element in my ongoing healing journey – it may or not be for you.*

5-MeO-DMT is found in a wide variety of plant species, and also is secreted by the glands of at least one toad species, the Colorado River toad[1]. Like its close relatives DMT[2] and bufotenin[3] (5-HO-DMT), it has been used as an entheogen[4] in South America[5]. Slang terms include Five-methoxy, the power, bufo, the God molecule, and toad venom.

The first time I heard about 5-MeO-DMT (5-MeO) I was kind of turned off and had no intention of using it. Anne-Marie, my God-sent therapist, had connected me to Mark, who had a similar story to mine. He exuberantly shared how his life had been changed by 5-MeO:

"They call it the businessman's psychedelic. You can make an appointment for 10:00 in the morning - be in and out in an hour – no major prep, no ceremony – and back to work after lunch. It was amazing!"

He couldn't recommend it highly enough, but to me it sounded too much like a silver bullet or a medicinal cure. It sounded too good to be true, and this was the first time I was hearing about it. Additionally, at that time I was in a months-long period of stability and, for the most part, symptom free.

A few months later I got an interesting voicemail from an old friend. "Hans! How are you doing? I'm just calling because I've come across an alternative medicine that has really helped me! Give me a call, I'd love to tell you about it."

Turns out, my friend's wife, who is from Mexico, had become trained to facilitate 5-MeO treatments. I began to do more research, talked with my therapist and reached out to other 5-MeO providers to get a better understanding of the medicine, the protocols, and whether it might be a fit for me.

Also, something I talk about elsewhere is taking the time to determine if this was indeed something that I was supposed to do; what was my motivation, did I feel pressured, afraid – was I manipulating things to make it happen? Was it aligning with my spiritual and intuitive journey, what did my close support people think? Was it falling into place naturally, or did it feel forced?

It took a couple of months before I felt I should move ahead, and to arrange the logistics. My friends live about 4 hours from me so I travelled to spend a few days with them. I was still somewhat hesitant and nervous but during the few days before, and also over the course of my weekend, some practical and personal details fell into place that felt like confirmation or direction that I was indeed on the right path – 5-MeO was meant to be part of my journey.

What was the actual medicine like? Not pleasant, not enjoyable, I didn't like the smell, the initial effect or the immediate after effect. Others have a different, more appealing experience. But for me, this is one of the clear cases where the lunacy of the common school of thought that psychedelics are similar to addictive drugs is apparent. There was absolutely no appeal or desire to take another dose of 5-MeO. Thirty seconds into the medicine session I wanted to quit. I had to be strongly encouraged to continue, and had to force myself to carry on with the protocol and take the recommended dose.

Unlike psilocybin and ayahuasca, the experience faded after 10 minutes, and within 45 minutes or so, I felt like I could carry on with normal conversation and activities. But, something had shifted.

For me it was subtle. Unlike the experience of others, I did not have a significant spiritual encounter or mental/emotional breakthrough. It wasn't until the next morning when I went for a walk that I was finally able to sense the gentle shift that had occurred; I felt like I had somehow moved forward. Something had been resolved from my past or a blockage removed that had prevented me from discovering my authentic self.

Interestingly, in the weeks and months that followed I was able to resolve some mental, emotional and relational issues that had pestered, no, actually tormented me for years. The shift was quite dramatic.

I am reluctant to point to 5-MeO, or any other particular modality as the only key to that period of breakthrough in my life. I was intensely practicing many other therapies, both conventional and alternative, in the months before and after my experience with this medicine. However, I am confident that it was a significant catalyst, and I am grateful for it.

PART SIX
CROSS-CULTURAL COMMUNICATION

CHAPTER 26
REMOVING BARRIERS

A shaman, a hippie and a yoga instructor walk into a bar...

One of my goals in writing this book is to increase awareness and accessibility to trauma therapy, somatics and psychedelics. I hope to remove obstacles and hindrances that prevent people who are trying to get better from trying new healing modalities.

One potential obstacle that I am aware of is related to the unique cultures associated with somatics and psychedelics. To start, some definitions:

Culture: The language, customs, arts, social institutions, and achievements of a particular nation, people, or other social group.

Cross-cultural communication: how people belonging to different cultures communicate with each other. It is communication between people who have differences in any one of the following: styles, worldviews, age, nationality, ethnicity, race, gender, sexual orientation, etc.

I have benefited extensively from the medical system in Canada. While active in injury-causing contact sports and other high-risk activities for decades, going through two surgeries for atrial fibrillation, and raising four boys, I have had countless visits to doctors and hospitals. During those interactions I have come to expect a certain style of communication, language and protocols. I think of this as the mainstream Western medical culture. This is the setting that most people in Canada are used to and comfortable with when they seek help for health issues. Most of us don't think about it or analyze it; in fact we don't necessarily even notice that we operate within a particular cultural context when we seek health care.

Similarly, most of us who have lived in Canada for most of our lives don't think about our national culture until we visit another country with different language, foods, and traditions.

I sincerely hope to be respectful of cultural identities and have due regard for the practices and traditions that need to remain tied to a particular ethnic group, religion, spiritual practice or cultural identity. However, where some of the elements and practices of somatics and psychedelics can be translated into the culture of Western medicine, I think it may be helpful to make that effort.

I am aware that some psychedelic ceremonies and somatic practices are rooted in the culture and spirituality of certain people groups and I am not suggesting that those be ignored or cast aside. On the contrary, at times, being open to and immersing myself in the spirituality and culture related to a particular plant medicine or somatic practice has been essential to my healing journey. I found it enriching and illuminating - I couldn't have moved forward in my healing without the cultural context and spirituality of some practices.

But where possible, I suggest that it could be helpful to either make more effort to communicate across cultures, or remove faux-culture barriers.

CHAPTER 27

MAXIMIZING ACCESSIBILITY TO PSYCHEDELICS

The first time I visited a therapist who was trained in psilocybin-assisted therapy he sat cross legged on the floor on a tie-dyed blanket while incense burned on a side table. No problem, I can roll with that. For me it wasn't off-putting, but for some who judge what lies ahead based on first impressions, it may seem quirky.

When I began exploring psilocybin-assisted therapy I soon came across words and phrases that puzzled me:

- Psychonaut
- Trip
- Tripping balls
- The mushroom spirit
- What is the mushroom saying to you?

Let's look at the word "trip." This word does not appeal to those with an aversion to the recreational drug scene, or those with a background in addiction. I was recently sharing with a friend who has a relative struggling with addiction about the ever-increasing use of psychedelics and he responded with, "I don't believe in people doing drugs to get off drugs."

How strange and unfortunate that many view psychedelics and other plant medicines as part of the nefarious addictive drug culture. Rather than "trip" I prefer the phrases "medicine session," or "psilocybin-assisted therapy session". I know this unfortunately adds a mouthful of additional syllables.

Here is a more innocuous example, but one that I find interesting. Recently I watched a lecture on psilocybin by an academic who delivered scholastic material in a professional manner - but was wearing a shirt covered with images of colorful little mushrooms. Cute, I guess, but kind of odd. Would an academic giving a lecture on anesthesiology wear a shirt with poppy flowers on it? I doubt it. If our goal is to attract people to alternative modalities, then removing these quirky cultural trip-lines may be prudent.

Most of us are very aware that psychedelics were being researched and utilized for mental health in the middle of the last century but were by-catch in Nixon's war on drugs and tragically grouped in with addictive narcotics and therefore restricted for decades. This was partly due to the hippie culture's use of psychedelics along with other more harmful drugs.

Unfortunately the stigma and stereotyping that pushed psychedelics away from adoption into mainstream medical practice is still among us today. I suggest we can learn from the past and do our utmost to pull these helpful and at times life-saving medicines into the context and culture of Western medicine.

As author Michael Pollan states in the film series *How to Change Your Mind*:

"We have to think about these substances in a very clear-eyed way, throw out the inherited thinking about it and, like, what is it good for? What if mental health problems like PTSD, OCD, alcoholism and depression could all be helped by psychoactive substances such as mescaline, psilocybin, MDMA, and even LSD?"

Words like "trip" and "psychonaut" are off putting to others as well. After a lifetime within the Western medical system, those willing to explore new and alternative modalities like somatics and psychedelics should not be burdened with the additional baggage of language carrying connotations of questionable value.

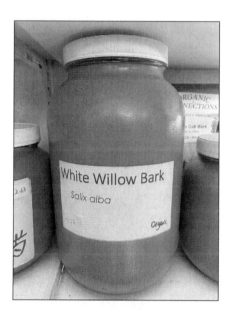

A full 40% of the drugs behind the pharmacist's counter in the Western world are derived from plants that people have used for centuries, including the top 20 best selling prescription drugs in North America today.

The humble aspirin is a modern miracle medicine and one of the most widely used drugs in the world. It's extracted from the bark of the willow tree, which was recommended for the treatment of aches and pains by the ancient Egyptians in the Ebers Papyrus. People used to chew twigs or make tea to alleviate pain and it's still possible to buy willow bark for this purpose. However, we never refer to aspirin as magic willow.

I prefer to use the word psilocybin rather than mushroom or

magic mushroom. I'm not dogmatic about it, but I find it to be more inclusive.

Another thing I find puzzling about psilocybin is the practice of ceremony. Forty years ago my friends and I would skip school on a Friday afternoon to pick 'shrooms from a cow pasture, bring them to a party that night and we would all do a bunch. Obviously, this was not therapeutic treatment, but recreational use of the reckless teenage variety, and I don't recommend it. However, in those days there was absolutely no thought or ideas about ceremony and spirituality. Nor am I aware of any ancestral local indigenous ceremonies involving psilocybin.

However, as the therapeutic use of psilocybin has increased, a variety of ceremonies for psilocybin have emerged with spiritual elements and protocols. For those whose experience is enhanced by ceremony, I think that is wonderful - go for it. But if it is restrictive or off-putting for some, then we need to provide for a discussion and delivery model that is accessible to those most comfortable in our Western medical culture.

If a ceremony is authentic and enhances the therapy, great! But if it is fabricated or causes fear and hesitation then in the spirit of invitation, inclusivity and accessibility, I suggest we provide alternatives.

As I've mentioned elsewhere, I believe there are multiple pathways to healing, to the application of the concepts in this book, and within our lives in general. What works for one person may not work for another. Applying the multiple pathways principle to the subject at hand provides for generosity and accessibility.

Once again, I am not disparaging those who thrive within the "shroom/trip/psychonaut" lingo and culture. I roll with that gang regularly and have come to see first-hand how their lives have benefited from plant medicine. I hope that their preferred cultural and ceremonial contexts continue to flourish. However, I also hope that plant medicines become as attractive and accessible to as many others as possible in order to expand opportunities for healing and transformation and potentially to save lives.

CROSS-CULTURAL COMMUNICATION AND 5-METHOXY-*N,N*-DIMETHYLTRYPTAMIN

All medicines are chemicals or combinations of chemicals. If I told my friends and family that my health had improved after taking a new medication called 5-methoxy-N,N-dimethyltryptamin, they would probably be happy for me. Because it sounds like a traditional medicine or chemical compound it would not warrant any exceptional explanation or be a cause for concern.

However, if I told them I had smoked some toad venom, or *"smoked the toad"* as some say, they would be concerned, laugh or be very puzzled. More importantly, how many sufferers avoid helpful substances because of strange nick-names and off-putting connections?

5-MeO-DMT is an example of a substance (still illegal in Canada) that has helped me and many others, but remains cloistered behind the walls of slang, stigma and stereotypes. Separate from the need for research, due diligence and the long political road to legality, it would be helpful in the meantime if terminology, labeling and discussion could be brought into the conventional realm of us "normies".

"I am not a psychedelic evangelist", Gabor Maté states emphatically. Similarly, I am not a "Western culture only" evangelist nor a "non-ceremony" evangelist. But perhaps I am a "multiple pathways and maximum accessibility" evangelist. In order to create opportunity and invitation, we have to examine our terminology and practices to ensure they are inclusive.

CHAPTER 28
RESPECTING WHAT IS SACRED

Sometimes psychedelics should absolutely remain within an authentic cultural context. This is not only out of respect for the culture, but also perhaps to attain maximum effect and healing.

This idea is beautifully illustrated in Chapter 31 of Gabor Maté's *The Myth of Normal*. The chapter title is "Jesus in the Tipi: Psychedelics and Healing."

The first eight pages of this chapter provide a detailed account of Maté's experience surrounding one of the many ayahuasca retreats he has been involved in leading. It is apparent throughout this wonderful experience that the breakthrough in Maté's healing, and also the integrity and depth of the experience for other attendees could take place only within the elaborate and well-established cultural context. The work and guidance of the Shipibo shamans at the Temple of Light in Northeastern Peru was essential. Essential is an understatement.

I did my ayahuasca ceremony here in Canada, but it was still rich in many areas of cultural authenticity. Interestingly, although the leader was visiting from Ecuador and had been taught the ceremony by his grandparents, he preferred to be called a knowledge-keeper rather than a shaman. One of his assistants told me that the word shaman carried connotations that were not always helpful.

The ceremony was conducted in Spanish, via an interpreter, and with elaborate cultural and spiritual elements. Clothing, setting, lighting, posture, songs, prayers, chants, fasting, stories, purging protocols, other plant medicines - these all contributed to the experience.

I can't imagine, nor have I heard of, a more culturally authentic ayahuasca ceremony outside of the actual countries that ayahuasca is indigenous to. However, the expense of traveling to one of these on-the-land ceremonies would have prohibited me from taking the medicine. The blended Canadian-Ecuadorian cross-cultural delivery allowed me to experience the healing benefits of Madre Ayahuasca.

Again, sometimes cultural context, especially with respect to Indigenous or ancient practices is the only vehicle for communication and delivery. Other times, I would suggest that it is appropriate to make a medicine available within the context of the culture where it is most accessible to those needing it.

SAUNA VS SWEAT LODGE

Another illustration of cross-cultural diversity can be found in the practice of taking a sauna, as opposed to attending an Indigenous sweat lodge. I love having a sauna and built my own in my backyard. My Scandinavian ancestors have been enjoying saunas for many generations. In recent decades research has proven the health benefits of saunas and the physiology of this old practice and tradition. However, as far as I know the Nordic sauna that my relatives have enjoyed for generations did not involve spiritual or ceremonial elements. When I visited family in Norway, Sweden, Finland and Estonia the sauna was typically an after dinner social event accompanied by a cold beverage and followed by dessert. It was a light-hearted affair with lots of banter and laughter. A therapeutic and healing evening for sure, but not ceremoniously serious.

Conversely, I have had the privilege and honour of participating in Indigenous sweats which are carried out over many hours and are rich in protocols, rituals and spiritual practices. The days-long setting up of the lodge, the collecting of stones (grandparents), smoking and passing the pipe, and the burning of wood (also ancestors) follows a formal set of traditions passed from generation to generation. Elders observe and provide oversight and direction.

It is obvious that these two practices have something in common; the participant bathes in hot steam in an enclosed space. However, one is rich with cultural and spiritual significance while the other is mainly recreational and social. Both have benefits, but recognizing and appreciating the diversity and value of both is a representation of cross-cultural diversity and respect. Approaching an indigenous sweat lodge ceremony with the casual and informal style of a Nordic sauna would be inconsiderate and offensive.

Some practices and traditions need to be respected and retained. However, to know which is which, we must make the effort to recognize both the similarities and unique elements of various practices.

CHAPTER 29
CROSS-CULTURAL COMMUNICATION FOR SOMATICS

A simple working definition for somatics that was conveyed to me is "mindful physical movement or body-based actions to release stress and trauma." As I suggested in the previous discussion involving psychedelics, it is sometimes essential that somatics be practiced within a cultural or spiritual context.

Research has proven the effectiveness of yoga as a somatic practice. I resisted yoga for years and stuck with other sports and exercises that I was used to. But over the last year, based on the advice of therapists and the writings of Maté, van der Kolk, Levine and others I have embraced the practice and really enjoy it.

Sometimes at the end of a class the instructor will express gratitude for a number of things including, "those in India who centuries ago developed these spiritual practices".

I have utmost respect for this idea and honour the history and tradition of yoga. But tbh, as a 225 pound, stiff and old ex-rugby player, I struggle through the movements while remaining meditative and breathing correctly - and I have no clue what the Indian phrases and postures are that the instructor speaks of. However, after a year of practice, it has improved my physical and mental health, and I have had breakthroughs in resolving my trauma because of it.

I have no idea whether I am participating partially or completely in what the ancient Indian practitioners intended centuries ago. But I do know that my intentions are good, I am open-minded and non-judgemental, and I am "moving my body to facilitate healing".

I have some friends who are Christians. Nice, compassionate, accepting and tolerant people. They love yoga but are more comfortable with the words and traditions of their own faith. They are completely accepting and honouring of other religions but find it easiest and most convenient to combine yoga movements with the spirituality and ideas of the Divine that they are used to.

Is that going to work? Will it carry the same somatic and trauma-healing benefits of yoga in a pure Eastern-religious context? I'm not sure - but I don't see why not.

Again, I am promoting accessibility and diversity - multiple pathways. Research is proving that we can resolve our trauma through somatics - my goal is to promote as many entry points to these healing modalities as possible. I hope that the ancient authentic practice of yoga with all its rich components remains vibrant and continues to grow. But if those who are suffering can be helped through non-spiritual simple movements and other forms of compassionate guidance, then I think we should be open to that as well.

Something else I have noticed that illustrates the benefit of cross-cultural generosity is the overlap between various expressions of body-based healing modalities and spiritual practices. Many somatic experiencing movements and methodologies are similar to those of:

- Polyvagal Theory,
- Nervous System Regulation
- Hindu and Buddhist energy systems based on chakras
- Taoist Yin practices focused on meridians

Each tradition may use different language or have a different explanation for what is happening in the body, or why a particular movement is beneficial, but the commonalities are glaring. Obviously, the human body is basically the same in India, China or North America. IMHO no one tradition or modality is ultimately superior to another, nor are they mutually exclusive - they all have the capacity to complement each other.

Some simple examples of similarities between practices:

- EMDR eye movement, and eye movement for Vagus nerve stimulation
- Peter Levine's "vooo sound", and the "om" sound in Hindu tradition
- Sauna and Indigenous sweat lodge
- Cold immersion and Indigenous cold bath

Again, it is not my intent to disrespect anyone nor to trivialize spiritual practices. I recognize that many have practiced these sacred traditions and religions their whole lives and have devoted themselves to them. I am new to all of these practices and admittedly a bit naive. I am simply pointing out some general observations based on my superficial exposure in an effort to help those suffering find the pathway, or pathways, that help them to get better.

WHAT'S YOUR POINT?

I think my main points in this part are:

- There are multiple cultures and traditions related to psychedelics and somatics
- Generosity, humility and open-mindedness are good things
- If a cultural or spiritual element related to somatics or psychedelics is confusing or a hindrance for some then

let's make the effort to help people overcome these
hurdles
• Where appropriate, recognize and retain the integrity
and purity of cultural expressions

I sincerely hope that it is clear that I am opposed to cultural appropriation. The majority of my career has involved working towards reconciliation and decolonization with Canada's Indigenous people. It would be unfortunate, and tragic actually, if the ideas on these pages were misinterpreted or misapplied in a way that was detrimental, offensive or disrespectful to the culture and traditions of a people group.

What I am promoting is the creative, but respectful development of avenues and opportunities for those who need these exciting and alternative modalities.

As I mentioned elsewhere, Peter Levine came up with somatics after watching a polar bear shaking on an Animal Kingdom TV show. Francine Shapiro discovered EMDR while walking through a park.

A few decades after Levine and Shapiro's curiosity and simplistic musings, somatics has become a profound, vast field of scientific study, thought and practice. EMDR is now an evidence-based therapy practiced throughout the world.

Imaginatively stripping what we do of unnecessary packaging and pseudo-cultural trappings, and bringing things back to their simplest form, purpose and application can demystify them and make them more accessible and inviting. Perhaps I'm pushing the envelope, but the goal is to relieve suffering and make people's lives better. In many cases, these tools could be not only life-changing, but life-saving.

AFTERWORD

BURN THIS BOOK

Either somatics and psychedelics do help to heal trauma or they don't. If they don't work and we are being misled - then please burn this book, find an alternative approach, and pursue your healing elsewhere.

I have included some of my personal experiences with somatics and psychedelics but those accounts are merely anecdotal and subjective. I am happy to share that my personal health has improved dramatically and some significant issues have disappeared. While life still brings challenges, my personal health is pretty darn good. I am grateful for the opportunity to share some of the information that has helped me.

However, what the backbone of this book really comes down to is the credibility and integrity of the scientists, researchers and experts leading the way in these new and exciting fields. Are they peddlers of hope, or shyster salesmen? Are they telling us the truth or selling us snake oil?

I believe they are truth-tellers - men and women of integrity.

Beyond their academic and literary success, I believe they are caring and compassionate. They are good humans, motivated to help people get better.

These world-renowned trauma specialists have devoted their lives, put their reputations on the line, and offered some big ideas that are either fat with flatulence or pregnant with promise:

- Everybody has trauma
- Trauma is trapped in our bodies
- Healing is possible
- Somatics and psychedelics can facilitate healing.

For some of us, the risk of hope, and the uncertainty of experimentation are worth it.

Some words of hope from Peter Levine:

"Every trauma provides an opportunity for authentic transformation. ... If we let it, trauma has the power to rob our lives of vitality and destroy it. However, we can also use it for powerful self-renewal and transformation. Trauma resolved is a blessing from a greater power."

Don't be surprised when your life starts getting better. You deserve that.

NOTES

1. EVERYONE HAS TRAUMA

1. Gabor Maté, "Dr. Gabor Maté Answers the Question: Is Everyone Traumatized?" | A *Mindspace* Podcast Clip: https://www.youtube.com/watch?v=RqCuUIRCREg
2. Peter Levine, "Dr. Peter Levine on Working through a Personal Traumatic Experience" | PsychAlive: https://www.youtube.com/watch?v=9hP2KJ3UgDI&t=3s
3. Gabor Maté, "Dr. Gabor Maté on Trauma, Addiction, and Illness under Capitalism" | The Real News Network: https://therealnews.com/dr-gabor-mate-on-trauma-addiction-and-illness-under-capitalism

2. THE SYMPTOMS OF TRAUMA

1. Gabor Maté, "How Childhood Trauma Leads to Addiction" | *After Skool*: https://www.youtube.com/watch?v=BVg2bfqblGI
2. Sukie Baxter, "How To Release Trauma Stored In The Body" | Sukie Baxter - Whole Body Revolution: https://www.youtube.com/watch?v=WQumUZfwyEQ
3. Gabor Maté, "Dr. Gabor Maté on the Effects of Trauma During Pregnancy and Childhood on Human Development" | *Mindspace*: https://www.youtube.com/watch?v=EHbXogI36Ic
4. Gabor Maté, "Dr Gabor Maté: Transgenerational Trauma, Stressed Environment, and Child's Diagnosis | *IoPT Norway*: https://www.youtube.com/watch?v=a13rn8Cduc&list=PLtOjliXfqhHZo4LP4K6AqhasuvB6iBg5Z&index=7

3. TRAUMA IS STORED IN YOUR BODY

1. Peter Levine, "Peter Levine Demonstrates How Trauma Sticks in the Body" | *PESI*: https://www.youtube.com/watch?v=fiqosILHiJs
2. BioBeats, "How unprocessed trauma is stored in the body" | Medium.com: https://medium.com/@biobeats/how-unprocessed-trauma-is-stored-in-the-body-10222a76cbad
3. "Past trauma may haunt your future health" | Harvard Medical School: https://www.health.harvard.edu/diseases-and-conditions/past-trauma-may-haunt-your-future-health

4. FAMILY

1. Noah Kahan - Homesick (Official Lyric Video): https://www.youtube.com/watch?v=ip-dkLJyMLg
2. Alanis Morissette: "Ablaze": https://www.youtube.com/watch?v=Dn6IO78BmRM

5. INTERGENERATIONAL TRAUMA

1. Gabor Maté, "Dr Gabor Maté: Transgenerational Trauma, Stressed Environment, and Child's Diagnosis | IoPT Norway: https://www.youtube.com/watch?v=-a13rn8Cduc&list=PLtOjliXfqhHZo4LP4K6AqhasuvB6iBg5Z&index=7
2. "Cultivating Transgenerational Resilience: Healing Ancestral Trauma" | Dr. Arielle Schwartz: https://www.youtube.com/watch?v=fDOtw5plaKI

6. ADDICTION AND TRAUMA

1. Gabor Maté, "The REAL Cause Of Drug Addiction...And A Plant Medicine Solution" | YouRevolution: https://www.youtube.com/watch?v=ov-a1Se2dEs
2. "How Childhood Trauma Leads to Addiction - Gabor Maté" | After Skool: https://www.youtube.com/watch?v=BVg2bfqblGI

8. DON'T WORRY, IT WILL GET WORSE

1. Dr. Pooky Knightsmith, "EMDR: 3 things I wish I'd known before I started trauma therapy" | Pooky Knightsmith Mental Health: https://www.youtube.com/watch?v=YSIYpnh9xEQ
2. Peter Levine, "A Simple Exercise to Ease Despair with Peter Levine, PhD" | NICABM: https://www.youtube.com/watch?v=n1bPdbBF1Ck
3. Bessel van de Kolk, "Overcome Trauma With Yoga" | KripaluVideo: https://www.youtube.com/watch?v=MmKfzbHzm_s
4. "How Meditation May Make Nervous System Dysregulation Worse" - Jessica Maguire: https://www.youtube.com/watch?v=OOlbrEdzo7E&list=PLtOjliXfqhHYaCvP9oXWD8CNmPN6LxzpO
5. "Why We Can Get Overwhelmed When We Start Healing Our Trauma" - Irene Lyon: https://www.youtube.com/watch?v=3uRMJV7L7sQ&list=PLtOjliXfqhHYaCvP9oXWD8CNmPN6LxzpO&index=3

9. RELAPSE

1. "What to know about anxiety" | MedicalNewsToday: https://www.medicalnewstoday.com/articles/323454
2. "What is depression and what can I do about it?" | MedicalNewsToday: https://www.medicalnewstoday.com/articles/8933
3. "Why do I have a headache? Causes, types, and remedies" | MedicalNewsToday: https://www.medicalnewstoday.com/articles/73936
4. "What causes fatigue, and how can I treat it?" | MedicalNewsToday: https://www.medicalnewstoday.com/articles/248002

10. WHY IS THIS TAKING ... SO ... BLOODY ... LONG?

1. Colin Hay: "Waiting for My Real Life to Begin": https://www.youtube.com/watch?v=Ko5isS9JQKM
2. [Trauma Tip #6] How Long Does It Take to Heal Trauma? | Irene Lyons: https://www.youtube.com/watch?v=RlmQxctdWJI
3. "Gabor Maté on Psychedelics, Trauma and the Body (Part 5)" | How To Academy Mindset: https://www.youtube.com/watch?v=ZzigPsgf9m8
4. Colin Hay: "Waiting for My Real Life to Begin": https://www.youtube.com/watch?v=Ko5isS9JQKM&ab_channel=ColinHay-Topic

11. TOOLS TO MINIMIZE RETRAUMATIZATION

1. Peter Levine, "What is Pendulation in Somatic Experiencing® with Peter A Levine, PhD" | Somatic Experiencing International: https://www.youtube.com/watch?v=LiXOMLoDm68

12. YOU DON'T HAVE TO TALK ABOUT IT

1. Dr. Arielle Schwartz, "Cultivating Transgenerational Resilience: Healing Ancestral Trauma" | Dr. Arielle Schwartz: https://www.youtube.com/watch?v=fDOtw5plaKI
2. Anna Runkle, "Telling Your Story Just Might Be Retraumatizing You" | Crappy Childhood Fairy: https://www.youtube.com/watch?v=sLiKHfCzlGs&list=PLtOjliXfqhHZo4LP4K6AqhasuvB6iBg5Z&index=4&t=867s
3. Dr. Pooky Knightsmith, "EMDR: 3 Things I Wish I'd Known Before I Started Trauma Therapy" | Pooky Knightsmith Mental Health: https://www.youtube.com/watch?v=YSIYpnh9xEQ

4. Dr. David Berceli, "TRE: A Condensed Explanation." | David Berceli: https://www.youtube.com/watch?app=desktop&v=eQkwLrSxd5w

13. WELCOME TO AA

1. Emotional Blindness, "Alexithymia" | Psychology Today: https://www.psychologytoday.com/us/basics/alexithymia

15. TRY EVERYTHING/MULTIPLE PATHWAYS

1. Bessel van der Kolk, "The 7 Surprising Ways To Heal Trauma WITHOUT MEDICATION" | Dr Rangan Chatterjee: https://www.youtube.com/watch?v=lrOBHyDRS-c&t=1692s

16. SELF-COMPASSION

1. Dr. Kristin Neff, "The Space Between Self-Esteem and Self Compassion" | TEDxTalks: https://www.youtube.com/watch?v=IvtZBUSplr4
2. Bessel van der Kolk, "Bessel van der Kolk - Effective Methods for Treating Trauma"| meg-rottweil: https://www.youtube.com/watch?v=B6sAoMxbU5g
3. "How the body keeps the score on trauma" | Big Think+: https://www.youtube.com/watch?v=iTefkqYQz8g
4. "The Space Between Self-Esteem and Self Compassion: Kristin Neff at TEDxCentennialParkWomen"| TEDx Talks: https://www.youtube.com/watch?v=IvtZBUSplr4&t=535s
5. Kristin Neff's website, Self-Compassion.org
6. "Self-Compassion: An Antidote to Shame" | Christopher Germer, Ph.D.: https://www.youtube.com/watch?v=rTFN8t9SXiQ&t=1370s

18. HYPE OR HOPE? DO SOMATICS WORK?

1. "Gabor Maté - Trauma Is Not What Happens to You, It Is What Happens Inside You" | Skoll.org: https://www.youtube.com/watch?v=nmJOuTAko9g

19. VOOO, SPHINCTER CONTRACTIONS, AND EAR MASSAGE

1. Peter Levine, "A Simple Exercise to Ease Despair with Peter Levine, PhD" | *NICABM*: https://www.youtube.com/watch?v=n1bPdbBF1Ck&list=PLtOjli XfqhHa3RKsuUUUWziRR5wVOMV4O&index=9&t=61s
2. Deepak Chopra, "How to Stimulate Your Vagus Nerve and Why You Should Try It" | The Chopra Well: https://www.youtube.com/watch?v=pHurINrDNVo& list=PLtOjliXfqhHa3RKsuUUUWziRR5wVOMV4O&index=5
3. Susie Baxter, "Vagus Nerve Massage For Stress And Anxiety Relief" | Sukie Baxter - Whole Body Revolution: https://www.youtube.com/watch?v=LnV3Q2x Ib1U&list=PLtOjliXfqhHa3RKsuUUUWziRR5wVOMV4O&index=2&t=418s

20. THE SHAKING BEAR

1. Peter Levine, "Nature's Lessons in Healing Trauma: An Introduction to Somatic Experiencing" | Somatic Experiencing International : https://www.youtube.com/watch?v=nmJDkzDMllc&list=PLBX-ZFhRWOWIuo-oyhFaM89owjERNMrGl
2. "Can Psychedelics Help Us Release Trauma Through Shaking?" | Psychedelic.-Support: https://psychedelic.support/resources/somatic-therapy-psychedelics-release-trauma/
3. Emma McAdam, "How to Release Emotions Trapped in Your Body 10/30 How to Process Emotions Like Trauma and Anxiety" | Therapy in a Nutshell: https://www.youtube.com/watch?v=GZw8fRPK-8k

21. EMDR

1. Francine Shapiro, "EMDR interview Francine Shapiro" | VEN EMDR: https://www.youtube.com/watch?v=8GUd5hhnkVE&t=339s

22. INTERGENERATIONAL SOMATICS

1. "Ocean Therapy Has the Power to Heal the Mind and Body" | Medical.Bag.com: https://www.medicalbag.com/home/lifestyle/ocean-therapy-has-the-power-to-heal-the-mind-and-body/
2. Alanis Morissette and Peter Levine, "Episode 8 - Conversation with Alanis Morissette & Dr. Peter Levine" | Alanis Morissette: https://www.youtube.com/watch?v=wDKo9A49tRU&t=1s

23. ALL THE KING'S HORSES

1. "Hallucinogen" | Wikipedia: https://en.wikipedia.org/wiki/Hallucinogen
2. Michael Kissinger, "Psychedelics Revisited" | UVic News: https://www.uvic.ca/news/topics/2021+torch-psychedelics-revisited+news
3. Gabor Maté, "Gabor Maté on Psychedelics, Trauma and the Body (Part 5)" | How To Academy Mindset: https://www.youtube.com/watch?v=ZzigPsgf9m8
4. Bessel van der Kolk, "The 7 SURPRISING Ways To Heal Trauma WITHOUT MEDICATION | Dr. Bessel Van Der Kolk" | Dr. Rangan Chaterjee: https://www.youtube.com/watch?v=lrOBHyDRS-c&t=1692s
5. Anders Beatty, "The REAL Cause of Drug Addiction...And a Plant Medicine Solution" | *YouRevolution*: https://www.youtube.com/watch?v=ov-a1Se2dEs

25. MY EXPERIENCE WITH 5-MEO-DMT

1. "Colorado River toad" | Wikipedia: https://en.m.wikipedia.org/wiki/Colorado_River_toad
2. "N,N-Dimethyltryptamine" | Wikipedia: https://en.m.wikipedia.org/wiki/Dimethyltryptamine
3. "Bufotenin" | Wikipedia: https://en.m.wikipedia.org/wiki/Bufotenin
4. "Entheogen" | Wikipedia: https://en.m.wikipedia.org/wiki/Entheogen
5. "South America" | Wikipedia: https://en.m.wikipedia.org/wiki/South_America

ABOUT THE AUTHOR

Hans P. Anderssen was born and raised in the beautiful Canadian west coast city of Victoria. Hans loves spending time with his family, cold-dipping in the ocean, playing soccer and hiking. He has worked as a forester, pastor, and for the last 15 years in Indigenous reconciliation. *The Quiet Part Out Loud* is Hans' first book.

More resources and Hans' contact info can be found at:

Quietpartoutloud.ca

Manufactured by Amazon.ca
Acheson, AB

13112411R00109